Dosage Calculations for Nursing Students

Master Dosage Calculations in 24 Hours
the Safe and Easy Way Without Formulas

AUTHORS:

Bradley J Wojcik, PharmD

Chase Hassen

Disclaimer:

Although the author and publisher have made every effort to ensure that the information in this book was correct at press time, the author and publisher do not assume and hereby disclaim any liability to any party for any loss, damage, or disruption caused by errors or omissions, whether such errors or omissions result from negligence, accident, or any other cause.

This book is not intended as a substitute for the medical advice of physicians. The reader should regularly consult a physician in matters relating to his/her health and particularly with respect to any symptoms that may require diagnosis or medical attention.

All rights reserved. No part of this publication may be reproduced, distributed, or transmitted in any form or by any means, including photocopying, recording, or other electronic or mechanical methods, without the prior written permission of the publisher, except in the case of brief quotations embodied in critical reviews and certain other noncommercial uses permitted by copyright law.

NCLEX®, NCLEX®-RN, and NCLEX®-PN are registered trademarks of the National Council of State Boards of Nursing, Inc. They hold no affiliation with this product.

Some images within this book are either royalty-free images, used under license from their respective copyright holders, or images that are in the public domain.

© **Copyright 2018 by Chase Hassen & Bradley J Wojcik, PharmD. All rights reserved.**

First, I want to give you this FREE gift...

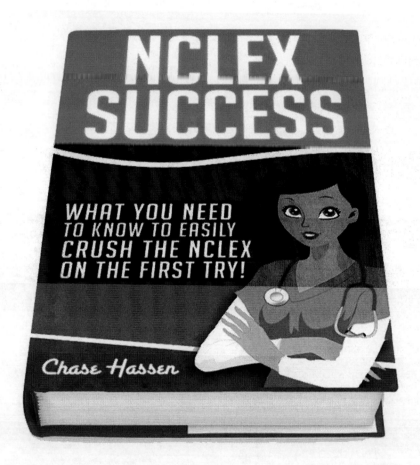

For a limited time, you can download this book for FREE.

Go To:

http://bit.ly/NCLEX2

Table of Contents

Introduction 7
    Unit 1: Essential Skills 9
Chapter 1 The Metric System 10
Chapter 2 Apothecary/Avoirdupois/Household Systems 12
Chapter 3 Ratios 13
    Tool Shed (Conversion Factors) 14
    Unit 2: Auxiliary Subjects 15
Chapter 4 Rounding Numbers 16
Chapter 5 Roman Numerals 18
    Roman Numeral Exercise 20
Chapter 6 Scientific Notation 23
    Scientific Notation Exercise 24
Chapter 7 Military Time (24-Hour Clock) 26
    Military Time Exercise 27
    Unit 3 Dimensional Analysis and Ratio Proportion 28
Chapter 8 Unit Conversions 32
    Unit Conversion Exercise using Dimensional Analysis 33
    Unit Conversion Exercise using Ratio Proportion 34
Chapter 9 Dosage Calculations 36
    Dosage Exercise Set 1 37
    Dosage Exercise Set 2 38
Chapter 10 IV Flow Rate Calculations 39
    IV Flow Rate Exercise 42
Chapter 11 Percent, Percent Strength, Ratio Strength 44
    Percent Exercise 46
    Percent Strength 48
    Percent Strength Exercise 49
    Ratio Strength 51
    Ratio Strength Exercise 52
Chapter 12 Milliequivalent Calculations 53
    Unit 4 Self-Assessment Exercise 57

Dosage Calculations for Nursing Students

Answers to Exercises 62

Military Time Exercise Answers 66

Dosage Exercise Set 1 Answers 69

Percent Change Exercise Answers 76

Percent Strength Exercise Answers 76

Milliequivalent Exercise Answers.. 79

Self-Assessment Exercise Answers... 82

Introduction

You are having some friends over for a BBQ and you will be grilling 24 hamburgers. You have plenty of hamburger patties, but you need 24 buns. You drive to the store and see that they are packaged 8 buns per package, so you pick up 3 packages. After getting home, you need to practice your dosage calculations and have the following problem. A provider has ordered 24 mg of a drug and you have on hand 8 mg/mL. How many mL will you administer? Did you need a hamburger bun formula to figure out how many packages of buns to buy? No, of course not, so why would you need a formula to calculate the dosage problem?

There are two main approaches to solving dosage calculations. You can either learn a long list of formulas, plug in the information from the problem and calculate the answer, or you can learn a few simple concepts and set up and solve the problem without resorting to formulas. This book takes the approach that it is safer and easier to learn what is happening in the problem and set up and solve it on your own.

Learning Objectives:

- The basics of the metric, apothecary, avoirdupois and household measurement systems.
- The three basic parts of dosage calculation problems.
- How to set up and solve dosage calculation problems using dimensional analysis.
- How to set up all calculations mathematically correct.
- Having enough confidence in your calculations skills to teach fellow students and maybe even your instructor.

What you will not learn:

- A long list of formulas.
- Moving the decimal point to the left or right.
- Multiplying or dividing by 1000, 30, 2.2 to convert units.
- Mathematically incorrect methods.

The book is divided into three main units followed by a self-assessment exercise.

Unit 1: Essential Skills:

You must know the basics of the metric system, apothecary, avoirdupois and household measurement systems to be successful in your calculations. Unit 1 also covers the basics of ratios, which form the foundation of dosage calculations.

Unit 2: Auxiliary Subjects:

Unit 2 covers rounding numbers, Roman numerals, scientific notation and military time. While rounding numbers could be considered an essential skill, the other subjects can probably be looked over briefly and returned to on an as needed basis.

Unit 3: Dimensional Analysis and Ratio Proportion:

Unit 3 is by far the most important unit in this book. All problems in this section can be solved using one easy method. Topics covered are:

- Dimensional Analysis vs. Ratio Proportion
- Unit Conversions
- Dosage Calculations
- IV Flow Rate Calculations
- Percent/Percent Strength/Ratio Strength Calculations
- Milliequivalent Calculations

Unit 4: Self-Assessment Exercise:

The book contains a self-assessment exercise which is broken into two parts: Part I contains problems which you must be able to do. Part II contains problems which you may not need for nursing but will be a good test for those of you who want to go above and beyond the basics.

General Terminology Used in this Book:

- **Number: Includes integers, decimal numbers, and fractions.**
    - Integer: All positive and negative whole numbers and zero.
        - ✓ Examples: -4, -3, 0, 2, 25
    - Decimal Number: A number which includes a decimal point.
        - ✓ Examples: 25.3, 0.05
    - Fraction: A number represented as a/b where a and b are both integers, with the exception that b cannot be 0.
        - ✓ Examples: 1/2, 3/4, 7/8, -1/2
- **Unit: Unit of measurement.**
    - Examples: mg, mL, kg, L.

A Few Important Notes:

- Always include all units of measurement (mg, g, L, mL, etc.) in the calculations.
    - The units are the most important part of the calculation. The numbers only go along for the ride.
- Set the calculations up mathematically correct.
    - 0.25 X 100% = 25% **not** 0.25 X 100 = 25%
- Use a space between the number and the unit.
    - 5 mL not 5mL
- Always use leading zeros on decimal numbers which are less than 1.

- > 0.5 mg not .5 mg.
- Always avoid trailing zeros after whole numbers.
  - > 5 mg not 5.0 mg
- Single quantities in equations can be expressed by themselves or as a ratio with 1 in the denominator. $2\text{ h}\left(\frac{60\text{ min}}{\text{h}}\right) = 120\text{ min}$ can be written $\frac{2\text{ h}}{1}\left(\frac{60\text{ min}}{\text{h}}\right) = 120\text{ min}$.
- Use mcg for microgram, not µg, as µg can be mistaken for mg.
- Definitions of terms in this book are limited in scope to the practice of pharmacy. You won't get a detailed technical definition of electrolytes, only that they are ions important to the function of the body.

Unit 1: Essential Skills

As with any subject, certain basic skills are required before delving into the actual subject matter. This book assumes that you know:

- Basic use of a simple calculator.
- Basic understanding of fractions and decimals.

Unit 1 covers:

- Basic units of the metric system used in nursing. You will be using these units every day in nursing school and on the job.
- Apothecary/Avoirdupois/Household Systems. These systems of measurement are used much less than the metric system, but it is still important to be familiar with them.
- Ratios. Virtually every dosage calculation, IV flow rate calculation and unit conversion will involve use of one or more ratios and it is vitally important that you fully understand them.

Chapter 1
The Metric System

- The metric system is the predominant system of measurement used in nursing.
- The primary base units used in nursing are gram, liter, and meter.
- Each of the base units can be multiplied or divided by powers of 10 to form larger or smaller units.
- Prefixes are placed before the base units to denote the larger and smaller units.
- The first table below lists the most important metric units used in nursing.

The Metric System Basics for Nurses

Prefix	Symbol	Multiple of base	Weight	Volume	Length
micro	mc	1/1,000,000	mcg		
mili	m	1/1000	mg	mL	mm
centi	c	1/100			cm
		Base Unit	g (gram)	L (liter)	m (meter)
kilo	k	1000	kg		km

Approximate Equivalents to Selected Metric Units

Weight Unit	Approximate Equivalent	Volume Unit	Approximate Equivalent	Length Unit	Approximate Equivalent
mcg	1 ant leg?	mL	20 drops	mm	1/25 inch
mg	6 grains of salt	L	1 quart	cm	4/10 inch
g	1 paperclip			m	1 yard
kg	2.2 lb			km	6/10 mile

Metric Prefixes Between 10^{18} and 10^{-18}

Prefix	Symbol	Multiplication Factor	Exponent
exa	E	1000000000000000000	10^{18}
peta	P	1000000000000000	10^{15}
tera	T	1000000000000	10^{12}
giga	G	1000000000	10^{9}
mega	M	1000000	10^{6}
kilo	k	1000	10^{3}
hecto	h	100	10^{2}
deca	da	10	10^{1}
	Base Unit	1	10^{0}
deci	d	0.1	10^{-1}
centi	c	0.01	10^{-2}
milli	m	0.001	10^{-3}
micro	mc	0.000001	10^{-6}
nano	n	0.000000001	10^{-9}
pico	p	0.000000000001	10^{-12}
femto	f	0.000000000000001	10^{-15}
atto	a	0.000000000000000001	10^{-18}

It is essential that you know the following equivalences. If you run into other units such as dL, you can always reference the above chart.

- 1 kg = 1000 g
- 1 g = 1000 mg
- 1 mg = 1000 mcg
- 1 L = 1000 mL
- 1 m = 100 cm
- 1 cm = 10 mm

These equations will form the basis for the ratios which you will learn about in Chapter 3.

Chapter 2
Apothecary/Avoirdupois/Household Systems

- These systems are rarely used in nursing today, but there are a few units and key points which should be learned.
- **Weight Units:**
    - Grain (gr): Technically 64.8 mg, but usually rounded to 65 mg.
    - Ounce (oz): Technically 28.3 g, but usually rounded to 30 g.
    - Pound (lb): Contains 16 oz. Usually rounded to 454 g.
- **Volume Units:**
    - Fluidram/fluid dram: Technically 3.7 mL, but usually rounded to 5 mL.
    - Fluid ounce: Technically 29.6 mL, but usually rounded to 30 mL.
    - Pint: 16 fluid ounces. Technically 473 mL, but usually rounded to 480 mL.
    - Teaspoonful: 5 mL
    - Tablespoonful: 15 mL

Important Units with Rounded Metric Equivalents

Apothecary Volume	Household Volume	Metric Volume
1 fluidram /fluid dram	1 teaspoonful (tsp)	5 mL
1 fluid ounce	2 tablespoonfuls (tbs)	30 mL
16 fluid ounces	1 pint (pt)	480 mL (473 mL)
	1 tablespoonful	15 mL
Apothecary Weight		**Metric Weight**
1 grain (gr)		65 mg
Avoirdupois Weight	**Household Weight**	**Metric Weight**
1 ounce (oz)	1 ounce (oz)	30 g
1 pound (lb)	1 pound (lb)	454 g (0.454 kg)

It is important that you know the following equivalences.

- 1 tsp = 5 mL
- 1 fl oz = 30 mL
- 1 gr = 65 mg
- 1 lb = 454 g
- 1 kg = 2.2 lb
- 1 lb = 16 oz

Chapter 3
Ratios

If you Google "ratios" you will see a lot of different definitions. What we will be dealing with in this book is dimensioned ratios, that is ratios which have units of measurement attached. These ratios are the foundation of the calculations you will learn in this book.

In Chapter 1 and 2 you were asked to learn the following equivalences:

- 1 kg = 1000 g
- 1 g = 1000 mg
- 1 mg = 1000 mcg
- 1 L = 1000 mL
- 1 m = 100 cm
- 1 cm = 10 mm
- 1 tsp = 5 mL
- 1 fl oz = 30 mL
- 1 gr = 65 mg
- 1 lb = 454 g
- 1 kg = 2.2 lb
- 1 lb = 16 oz

Looking at 1 kg = 1000 g, we can say that there are 1000 g per 1 kg. This can be written:

$$\frac{1000 \text{ g}}{1 \text{ kg}}$$

You could also say that there is 1 kg per 1000 g and write:

$$\frac{1 \text{ kg}}{1000 \text{ g}}$$

Here is the fun part. 1 kg = 1000 g and 5 = 5. Just like $\frac{5}{5} = 1$, $\frac{1 \text{ kg}}{1000 \text{ g}} = 1$!

Why is it important to know that $\frac{1 \text{ kg}}{1000 \text{ g}} = 1$? Because we can multiply anything by 1 or a form of 1 and not change its value. If you are asked to calculate the number of kg in 5200 g, you can simply multiply 5200 g by $\frac{1 \text{ kg}}{1000 \text{ g}}$. The g's will cancel out giving you 5.2 kg. Think of the ratios as tools which are used to change the units of what you are given into the units of the answer. The following chart contains a list of ratios (conversion factors) you can use in your calculations.

Tool Shed (Conversion Factors)

These conversion factors equal 1 and can be flipped upside down, if needed.

Metric Weight: $\left(\frac{1\text{ g}}{1000\text{ mg}}\right)\left(\frac{1000\text{ mg}}{1\text{ g}}\right)\left(\frac{1\text{ kg}}{1000\text{ g}}\right)\left(\frac{1000\text{ g}}{1\text{ kg}}\right)\left(\frac{1\text{ mg}}{1000\text{ mcg}}\right)\left(\frac{1000\text{ mcg}}{1\text{ mg}}\right)$

Metric Volume: $\left(\frac{1\text{ L}}{1000\text{ mL}}\right)\left(\frac{1000\text{ mL}}{1\text{ L}}\right)$

Metric - U.S Weight: $\left(\frac{30\text{ g}}{1\text{ oz}}\right)\left(\frac{1\text{ oz}}{30\text{ g}}\right)\left(\frac{2.2\text{ lb}}{1\text{ kg}}\right)\left(\frac{1\text{ kg}}{2.2\text{ lb}}\right)\left(\frac{1\text{ lb}}{454\text{ g}}\right)\left(\frac{454\text{ g}}{1\text{ lb}}\right)$

Metric – US Volume: $\left(\frac{1\text{ tsp}}{5\text{ mL}}\right)\left(\frac{5\text{ mL}}{1\text{ tsp}}\right)\left(\frac{1\text{ oz}}{30\text{ mL}}\right)\left(\frac{30\text{ mL}}{1\text{ oz}}\right)\left(\frac{1\text{ pt}}{480\text{ mL}}\right)\left(\frac{480\text{ mL}}{1\text{ pt}}\right)\left(\frac{1\text{ tbs}}{15\text{ mL}}\right)\left(\frac{15\text{ mL}}{1\text{ tbs}}\right)$

U.S. Volume: $\left(\frac{1\text{ tbs}}{3\text{ tsp}}\right)\left(\frac{3\text{ tsp}}{1\text{ tbs}}\right)\left(\frac{16\text{ oz}}{1\text{ pt}}\right)\left(\frac{1\text{ pt}}{16\text{ oz}}\right)\left(\frac{1\text{ qt}}{2\text{ pt}}\right)\left(\frac{8\text{ oz}}{1\text{ cup}}\right)\left(\frac{1\text{ cup}}{8\text{ oz}}\right)\left(\frac{1\text{ gal}}{4\text{ qt}}\right)\left(\frac{4\text{ qt}}{1\text{ gal}}\right)$

Metric Length: $\left(\frac{1\text{ m}}{100\text{ cm}}\right)\left(\frac{100\text{ cm}}{1\text{ m}}\right)\left(\frac{1\text{ cm}}{10\text{ mm}}\right)\left(\frac{10\text{ mm}}{1\text{ cm}}\right)$

Metric - U.S. Length: $\left(\frac{1\text{ in}}{2.54\text{ cm}}\right)\left(\frac{2.54\text{ cm}}{1\text{ in}}\right)$

Apothecary - Metric Volume: $\left(\frac{1\text{ fl dram}}{5\text{ mL}}\right)\left(\frac{5\text{ mL}}{1\text{ fl dram}}\right)\left(\frac{1\text{ fl oz}}{30\text{ mL}}\right)\left(\frac{30\text{ mL}}{1\text{ fl oz}}\right)$

Apothecary - Metric Weight: $\left(\frac{65\text{ mg}}{1\text{ gr}}\right)\left(\frac{1\text{ gr}}{65\text{ mg}}\right)$

Percent: $\left(\frac{1}{100\%}\right)\left(\frac{100\%}{1}\right)(100\%)$

Time: $\left(\frac{60\text{ sec}}{\text{min}}\right)\left(\frac{1\text{ min}}{60\text{ sec}}\right)\left(\frac{60\text{ min}}{\text{h}}\right)\left(\frac{1\text{ h}}{60\text{ min}}\right)\left(\frac{24\text{ h}}{\text{d}}\right)\left(\frac{1\text{ d}}{24\text{ h}}\right)$

Temperature: °F = (1.8 °C) + 32°

What about all the other ratios you encounter in dosage calculations? How about that bottle of amoxicillin 250 mg/5 mL you have in the refrigerator? Does 250 mg = 5 mL and $\frac{250\text{ mg}}{5\text{ mL}} = 1$? Yes, if a ratio is given to you in a problem, it will equal 1. The patient will receive the same amount of amoxicillin weather 250 mg or 5 mL of the suspension is administered.

Summary

All the conversion factors listed in the Tool Shed always hold true and can be used whenever needed. All conversion factors can be flipped upside down if need and they always equal 1.

All ratios given in a dosage problem equal 1 and can be flipped upside down if needed. Examples include drug strengths (100 mg/1 mL, 500 mg/ 1 tablet) drop factors (15 drops/ 1 mL) weight-based dosages (10 mg/kg).

Unit 3 will go into detail on how to put your knowledge of ratios to work solving problems. Understanding the information in this unit is half the battle. The rest is easy.

Unit 2: Auxiliary Subjects

Unit 2 covers topics which are helpful but may not be used extensively in nursing calculations. You can either study these topics now or come back to them if needed.

Topics covered in Unit 2:

- Rounding Numbers
- Roman Numerals
- Scientific Notation
- Basic Percent Calculations
- Military Time

Chapter 4
Rounding Numbers

Many times, calculated answers will have more decimal places than needed or desired and rounding will be required. To round a number:

- Identify the digit occupying the place to be rounded to. For example, if asked to round to the nearest tenth, you would look at the 8 in the following example.

3	5	6	.	8	1	9
Hundreds	Tens	Ones	Decimal Point	Tenths	Hundredths	Thousandths

- Look at the digit following the digit being rounded. In the above example, this is the 1.
- If the following digit is 0,1,2,3, or 4, all digits following the digit being rounded are dropped and you are finished. In the above example, the 1 and 9 are dropped, leaving 356.8 as the rounded number.
- If the following digit is 5,6,7,8, or 9, all digits following the digit being rounded are dropped, and the digit is increase by 1. In rounding the number 156.879 to the nearest tenth, the 7 and 9 are dropped and the 8 is increased to 9, leaving 156.9 as the rounded number.

IMPORTANT: When rounding numbers, look ONLY at the first digit after the digit being rounded. All other digits are irrelevant.

Example: Round to the nearest tenth.

- 6.759 rounded is 6.8 (Look only at the 5; the 9 is irrelevant.)
- 10.248 rounded is 10.2 (Look only at the 4; the 8 is irrelevant.)
- 0.38999 rounded is 0.4 (Look only at the 8; the 9's are irrelevant.)

Example: Round to the nearest hundredth.

- 89.523 rounded is 89.52
- 0.59788 rounded is 0.60
- 7.2395 rounded is 7.24

Rounding Exercise

	Round to the Nearest Tenth	Rounded Number		Round to the Nearest Hundredth	Rounded Number
1	6.88	6.9	26	89.568	89.57
2	7.54		27	45.789	
3	2.22		28	1.005	
4	3.08		29	2.895	
5	78.53		30	3.997	
6	99.23		31	7.894	
7	101.16		32	3.433	
8	5.44		33	2.222	
9	99.99		34	1.111	
10	53.247		35	8.895	
11	9.355		36	3.578	
12	100.01		37	2.2256	
13	56.3756		38	90.3895	
14	9.56		39	78.451	
15	22.56		40	3.215	
16	78.59		41	9.782	
17	77.459		42	10.554	
18	3.57		43	3.987	
19	9.78		44	1.9954	
20	23.598		45	2.493	
21	78.3		46	8.523	
22	78.303		47	9.672	
23	798.32		48	4.956	
24	8.06		49	2.225	
25	9.11		50	3.987	

Chapter 5
Roman Numerals

- **The decimal number system, also called the Arabic number system, is a positional number system in which the position of the digit determines its value. The 2 in 521 represents 20, but the 2 in 245 represents 200.**
- **The Roman numeral system is an additive and subtractive system in which the value of a numeral remains constant. The C in CXX represents a value of 100, just as the C in CLXV represents 100.**

Roman Numerals and Their Values

Roman Numeral	Value	Memory Hints
SS	1/2	Short stack of pancakes, which is about half a regular stack.
I	1	Easy to remember because it looks like a 1.
V	5	Your hand with your fingers together and thumb apart forms a V.
X	10	Think of it as two V's, one on top of the other.
L	50	Think of **L**asso. It has 5 letters and ends in O (50).
C	100	Think of **C**entury or **C**-note.
D	500	Imagine 500 **D**ogs in your house, all barking and running around.
M	1000	Think of **M**illennium.

Rules for Forming Roman Numerals

1) Start from the left with the largest numeral and work down to the smallest on the right.

2) No more than three of the same numeral in a row. 40 cannot be written XXXX.

3) If a smaller numeral is placed before a larger numeral, the smaller numeral is subtracted from the larger numeral. For example, IV is 4; the I is subtracted from V (5-1).

4) Only I, X, and C may be subtracted from a larger numeral. The "five" numerals (V, L, D) may not be subtracted from a larger numeral. 45 is written XLV, not VL.

5) When a smaller numeral is subtracted from a larger numeral, the smaller numeral can be no less than one tenth of the larger numeral. IX is 9, but IL is not permitted for 49, nor IC for 99. 49 is written XLIX and 99 is written XCIX. Only one numeral at a time may be subtracted and only from one other numeral. IIX is not permitted for 8, nor IXX for 19.

6) Always use the largest numerals possible. 15 is written XV, not VVV, even though writing three V's does not break rule #2.

These rules may seem complicated, but with a little practice Roman numerals are easy if you learn the following tips.

- A smaller numeral must be subtracted from a larger numeral only if the number contains a 4 or 9. 246 is written CCXLVI with the X being subtracted from the L. 2386 is written MMCCCLXXXVI, with no subtraction involved.
- When one numeral is subtracted from another, think of them as a unit. Think of IV as 4, not 5-1, XL as 40, not 50-10, etc.
- Learn the following table to be able to quickly form any Roman numeral.

1000	M	100	C	10	X	1	I
2000	MM	200	CC	20	XX	2	II
3000	MMM	300	CCC	30	XXX	3	III
		400	CD	40	XL	4	IV
		500	D	50	L	5	V
		600	DC	60	LX	6	VI
		700	DCC	70	LXX	7	VII
		800	DCCC	80	LXXX	8	VIII
		900	CM	90	XC	9	IX
						1/2	SS

Example: Convert 2648 to a Roman numeral.

- Separate out the 1000's, 100's, 10's, and 1's and place the corresponding Roman numeral next to them.

2000	MM
600	DC
40	XL
8	VIII

- Line up the Roman numerals in order starting with the largest.
  - ➢ MMDCXLVIII

Example: Convert MCMXXXIV to a number.

- Separate out the 1000's, 100's, 10's, and 1's and place the corresponding number next to them.

M	1000
CM	900
XXX	30
IV	4

- Total the numbers.
  - ➢ 1934

Roman Numeral Exercise

1) You must know the eight basic Roman numerals and their number counterparts:

SS, I, V, X, L, C, D, M. Fill in the blanks in the following tables.

Roman Numeral	Number
SS	
I	
V	
X	
L	
C	
D	
M	

Number	Roman Numeral
1/2 (0.5)	
1	
5	
10	

50	
100	
500	
1000	

2) Fill in the blanks with the corresponding Roman numerals or numbers.

50		C	
100		5	
1/2		10	
X		L	
M		I	
5		X	
V		D	
500		M	
L		X	
SS		V	
1000		L	
1		C	
D		5	
L		50	
M		1000	
10		100	

3) Fill in the blanks with the corresponding Roman numerals.

1000		100		10		1	
2000		200		20		2	
3000		300		30		3	
		400		40		4	
		500		50		5	
		600		60		6	
		700		70		7	
		800		80		8	
		900		90		9	
						1/2	

Dosage Calculations for Nursing Students

4) Fill in the blanks with the corresponding number or Roman numeral.

10		LXX	
30		20	
400		CCC	
DC		CD	
2000		CM	
8		700	
XC		50	
40		20	
60		LXXX	
200		DCC	
900		600	
IV		CC	
III		9	
SS		4	

5) Write the corresponding Roman numerals or numbers:

Example: Write 2782 as a Roman numeral.

2000	MM
700	DCC
80	LXXX
2	II

- **Line up the Roman numerals in order starting with the largest.**
  - MMDCCLXXXII

Example: Write MMDCLXXVI as a number.

MM	2000
DC	600
LXX	70
VI	6

- **Total the numbers.**
  - 2676

22 | Page

Chapter 6
Scientific Notation

- **Scientific notation is an easier way to write very large and very small numbers.**
- Example: 602,200,000,000,000,000,000,000 becomes 6.022 X 10^{23} in scientific notation.
- Example: 0.00000000000000000019942 becomes 1.9942 X 10^{-18} in scientific notation.

Terminology:
- **Exponent:** The small number written just above and to the right of a base number. It is the 23 in 6.022 X 10^{23} and denotes the number of times 10 is used in a multiplication.
  - 10^2 denotes 10 X 10. 10^3 denotes 10 X 10 X 10.
  - A negative exponent denotes 1 divided by the 10's, which results in a number less than 1. For example, 10^{-2} is $1/10^2$, or 1/100, which is 0.01.
- **Coefficient:** The number which is multiplied by 10 raised to the exponent. It is the 6.022 in 6.022 X 10^{23}. It is always at least 1 and less than 10.

Steps to Write a Number in Scientific Notation

Examples using 6,154,000,000 and 0.000816:

Step 1) Separate out the digits which are either before or after all the zeros and place a decimal point after the first digit, forming the coefficient.
- 6,154,000,000:   6.154
- 0.000816:   8.16

Step 2) Look at the original number and count the number of places to move the decimal point either to the end or back to the original decimal point from the decimal point in the coefficient.

- **6,154,000,000: 9 places from between the 6 & 1 to the end.**
- **0.000816: 4 places back from between the 8 & 1 to the original decimal point.**

Step 3) Write the coefficient and multiply it by 10 raised to the number of places the decimal point was moved. If the decimal point was moved to the right, the exponent is positive; if the decimal point was moved to the left, the exponent is negative.

Dosage Calculations for Nursing Students

- **6.154 X 10^9**
- **8.16 X 10^{-4}**

Examples:

Number	Scientific Notation
5,015,000	5.015 X 10^6
3,000	3 X 10^3
645,000,000	6.45 X 10^8
0.00056	5.6 X 10^{-4}
0.00000734	7.34 X 10^{-6}
0.00003005	3.005 X 10^{-5}

Scientific Notation Exercise

1) Convert the following numbers to scientific notation.

Number	Coefficient	# of Places from New Decimal Point to end of Original Number	Coefficient X 10 Raised to the Number of Places the Decimal Point was Moved
67,000	6.7	4	**6.7 X 10^4**
2,387,000	2.387	6	**2.387 X 10^6**
7,000,000			
98,000			
432,000,000			
900,000,000			
58,000,000,000			
2,478,000,000			
92,000,000			
60,230,000,000			
105,000			

2) Convert the following decimal numbers to scientific notation.

Decimal Number	Coefficient	# of Places from New Decimal Point to Original Decimal Point	Coefficient X 10 Raised to the Negative Number of Places the Decimal Point was Moved
0.056	5.6	2	**5.6 X 10^{-2}**
0.000380	3.80	4	**3.80 X 10^{-4}**
0.00007			
0.00002039			
0.0005078			
0.00001832			
0.000650			
0.0000000012			
0.000054			
0.000783			
0.00034			

3) Convert the following numbers from scientific notation to numbers.

Scientific Notation	Coefficient	Exponent	# of Places to Move the Decimal Point to the Right	Number
5.62×10^6	5.62	6	6	5,620,000
7.8×10^7	7.8	7	7	78,000,000
9×10^5	9	5	5	900,000
6.02×10^7	6.02	7	7	60,200,000
1.05×10^4	1.05	4	4	10,500
9.78×10^9	9.78	9	9	9,780,000,000
6.99×10^3	6.99	3	3	6,990
3.78×10^8	3.78	8	8	378,000,000
4.0×10^8	4.0	8	8	400,000,000
7.66×10^5	7.66	5	5	766,000

4) Convert the following decimal numbers from scientific notation to decimal numbers.

Scientific Notation	Coefficient	Exponent	# of Places to Move the Decimal Point to the Left	Decimal Number
6.05×10^{-4}	6.05	-4	4	0.000605
2.3×10^{-7}	2.3	-7	7	0.00000023
7.80×10^{-4}	7.80	-4	4	0.000780
3.5×10^{-6}	3.5	-6	6	0.0000035
8.995×10^{-5}	8.995	-5	5	0.00008995
1.023×10^{-9}	1.023	-9	9	0.000000001023
5.00×10^{-4}	5.00	-4	4	0.000500
8.43×10^{-6}	8.43	-6	6	0.00000843
2.22×10^{-3}	2.22	-3	3	0.00222
1.6×10^{-7}	1.6	-7	7	0.00000016

Chapter 7
Military Time (24-Hour Clock)

Hospitals typically use military time rather than civilian time (12 hour-a.m./p.m.).

- Military time is based on a 24-hour clock.
- The following chart gives the corresponding military times and civilian times.
- The times between 1:00 AM and 12:59 PM are the same in military time as they are in civilian time. Just remove the colon and add a zero in front of the numbers below 10.
- For times between 1:00 PM and 11:59 PM, add 12 hours to convert to military time.
- For times between 12:00 Midnight and 12:59 AM, subtract 12 hours.

Civilian Time	Military Time (24-Hour)	Civilian Time	Military Time (24-Hour)
Midnight	0000 or 2400	Noon	1200
12:01 AM	0001	12:01 PM	1201
1:00 AM	0100	1:00 PM	1300
2:00 AM	0200	2:00 PM	1400
3:00 AM	0300	3:00 PM	1500
4:00 AM	0400	4:00 PM	1600
5:00 AM	0500	5:00 PM	1700
6:00 AM	0600	6:00 PM	1800
7:00 AM	0700	7:00 PM	1900
8:00 AM	0800	8:00 PM	2000
9:00 AM	0900	9:00 PM	2100
10:00 AM	1000	10:00 PM	2200
11:00 AM	1100	11:00 PM	2300

Military Time Exercise

Convert the following civilian times to military time.

1) 5:15 AM

2) 12:25 AM

3) 8:27 PM

4) 11:19 PM

5) 6:00 AM

Convert the following military times to civilian times.

6) 0520

7) 2301

8) 1205

9) 0610

10) 1301

11) You started work at 0600 and you ended work at 1400. You didn't get any lunch or breaks (poor you). How many hours did you work?

12) An IV was started at 1100 and ended at 2:30 PM. How many hours did it run?

13) You have the weekend off. You started watching your favorite Netflix series at 0730 on Saturday morning and finished at 0130 on Sunday. How many hours did you sit on the couch watching TV?

14) A patient is admitted at 0600 and pushes his call button 8 times between 0600 and 0616. What is the average time interval between button pushes?

Unit 3 Dimensional Analysis and Ratio Proportion

If you know the basics of the metric, apothecary, avoirdupois and household systems of measurements and you know that all the ratios you will be working with equal 1 and can be flipped upside down when needed, then you are ready to learn the most important unit in the book.

Terminology:

- **Dimensional Analysis (DA):** A powerful method of solving problems in nursing, pharmacy, chemistry, physics, and engineering in which a given is multiplied by one or more ratios to obtain the answer.
- **Ratio Proportion (RP):** A method widely used by the medical community to solve problems by comparing two ratios.

It is extremely important to fully understand everything in this chapter.

Most of the calculations encountered in nursing involve nothing more than changing the units from what is given to the units desired. These include:

- Unit Conversions
- Dosage Calculations
- IV Flow Rate Calculations
- Percent, Percent Strength, and Ratio Strength Calculations
- Milliequivalent Calculations

These calculations can all be solved using DA or RP.

Think of these not as five different types of calculations, but as a single type of calculation involving five different types of units.

These problems all have the same three parts:

- **The Units of the Answer:** Think of it as the destination.
- **A Given:** This is what is given to start the problem and what is changed into the answer.
- **One or More Ratios:** These are the tools used to change the units of the given into the units of the answer.

Example 1 using DA: Convert 4.5 g into mg.

- The units of the answer are mg. This is the destination.
- The given is 4.5 g. This is the starting point.
- The ratio is 1000 mg/g. This is the tool to change g to mg.
- Start by listing the starting point and destination. This will help when placing the ratio(s).

$$4.5 \text{ g} \quad = \quad \text{mg}$$

- Place the ratio with the units of the answer on top and the units to be canceled on the bottom. Multiply the given by the ratio. The grams cancel out, leaving mg in the answer.

$$4.5\ g\left(\frac{1000\ mg}{g}\right) = 4500\ mg \quad \text{or} \quad \frac{4.5\ g}{1}\left(\frac{1000\ mg}{g}\right) = 4500\ mg$$

Example 2 using DA: A patient is prescribed 400 mg. The drug is available in a strength of 200 mg/mL. How many mL will be administered?

- The units of the answer are mL.
- The given is 400 mg.
- The ratio is 200 mg/mL.
- Start by listing the starting point and destination.

$$400\ mg \quad - \quad mL$$

- Place the ratio with the units of the answer on top and the units to be canceled on the bottom. Multiply the given by the ratio. The mg cancel out leaving, leaving mL.

$$400\ mg\left(\frac{1\ mL}{200\ mg}\right) = 2\ mL$$

- In this case, the ratio was flipped upside down placing mL on top and mg on the bottom.

Key Points about the Ratios

- **The ratios always equal 1.** Since 1000 mg = 1 g, $\frac{1000\ mg}{1\ g} = 1$ (In this book, this type of ratio is called an "off the shelf" ratio because it is always true. There are always 1000 mg in a g.)
  In example 2, it is stated the drug's strength is 200 mg/mL. For this problem, it can be stated that 1 mL = 200 mg. $\frac{1\ mL}{200\ mg} = 1$ and $\frac{200\ mg}{1\ mL} = 1$. (In this book, this type of ratio is called a "custom ratio" because it only holds true for the problem at hand. There are not always 200 mg/mL, only if the problem states it.)
- **The ratios can be flipped upside down if needed.** $\frac{1000\ mg}{1\ g} = \frac{1\ g}{1000\ mg} = 1$

The above two examples were solved using the dimensional analysis method. An explanation of the ratio proportion method follows.

Dosage Calculations for Nursing Students

The Ratio Proportion Method

The ratio proportion method is the other method used to solve the problems in this unit. Using the ratio proportion method, also called the ratio and proportion method, two ratios are set up that are proportional (equal) to each other and the unknown is solved for. Using the above examples:

Example 1 using RP: Convert 4.5 g into mg.

- The RP method uses two ratios: one ratio containing the unknown and the given, the other ratio serving as a reference ratio.

$$\frac{x \text{ mg}}{4.5 \text{ g}} = \frac{1000 \text{ mg}}{1 \text{ g}}$$

- The easiest way to solve for x mg is to cross multiply (4.5 g)(1000 mg) then divide by 1 g, resulting in the answer of **4500 mg**.

Example 2 using RP: A patient is prescribed 400 mg. The drug is available in a strength of 200 mg/mL. How many mL will be administered?

$$\frac{x \text{ mL}}{400 \text{ mg}} = \frac{1 \text{ mL}}{200 \text{ mg}}$$

- **Solving for x mL: (400 mg)(1 mL)/200 mg = 2 mL**

When using the ratio proportion method, both numerators must have the same units and both denominators must have the same units.

For simple one step problems, there is not a lot of difference between DA and RP as far as ease of use or safety. Now consider the following problem, which involves several ratios, solved using both DA and RP.

Example 3 using DA: A 186 lb patient has been prescribed a dosage of 20 mg/kg. The drug is available in 10 mL vials each containing 2.5 g of drug. How many mL should be administered?

- The units of the answer are mL.
- The given is 186 lb.
- The ratios are 20 mg/kg, 2.5 g/10 mL, 2.2 lb/kg, 1000 mg/g.

$$186 \text{ lb} \left(\frac{1 \text{ kg}}{2.2 \text{ lb}}\right)\left(\frac{20 \text{ mg}}{\text{kg}}\right)\left(\frac{1 \text{ g}}{1000 \text{ mg}}\right)\left(\frac{10 \text{ mL}}{2.5 \text{ g}}\right) = 6.8 \text{ mL}$$

Example 3 using RP: A 186 lb patient has been prescribed a dosage of 20 mg/kg. The drug is available in 10 mL vials each containing 2.5 g of drug. How many mL should be administered?

- Step 1) Convert 186 lb to kg.

$$\frac{x \text{ kg}}{186 \text{ lb}} = \frac{1 \text{ kg}}{2.2 \text{ lb}}$$

  ➤ Solving for x kg yields 84.5 kg.

- Step 2) Calculate the dose of drug in mg needed for an 84.5 kg patient.

$$\frac{x\ mg}{84.5\ kg} = \frac{20\ mg}{kg}$$

> Solving for x mg yields 1690 mg
- Step 3) Convert 1690 mg to g.

$$\frac{x\ g}{1690\ mg} = \frac{1\ g}{1000\ mg}$$

> Solving for x g yields 1.69 g.
- Step 4) Calculate the dose in mL needed to deliver 1.69 g of drug.

$$\frac{x\ mL}{1.69\ g} = \frac{10\ mL}{2.5\ g}$$

> **Solving for x mL yields the answer: 6.8 mL.**

It is the authors' belief that the dimensional analysis method is superior to the ratio proportion method for problems involving more than one step.

- Using dimensional analysis, the problem can be set up in one step and checked for accuracy by canceling out the units before any calculations are performed.
- Using the ratio proportion method, several problems must be set up, complicating the problem and introducing sources of error.
- A small pile of gravel can be moved with an "RP shovel" but climb into a "DA bulldozer" to move a large pile.

Going forward, both the DA and RP method will be shown for the simple unit conversion problems, but only DA will be shown for the other problems.

Chapter 8
Unit Conversions

Terminology:

- **Unit:** Unit of measurement. The mg, g, mL, L, oz, kg, etc., that are used in nursing calculations.
- **Unit Conversions:** Converting from one unit to another without changing the value. If you don't remember all the conversion factors, refer to the tool shed in Chapter 3.

Using the Tools in the DA Method

- Write down the quantity to be converted on the left side of the equation, say 8.67 g, and the units of the answer on the right side of the equation, say mg.

$$8.67 \text{ g} = \quad \text{mg}$$

- Look in the tool shed for the tool (conversion factor) which has mg on top and g on the bottom. Under Metric Weight you will find $\left(\frac{1000 \text{ mg}}{\text{g}}\right)$.

- Place the tool to be used next to the quantity to be converted, cancel out the units, and multiply.

$$8.67 \text{g} \left(\frac{1000 \text{ mg}}{\text{g}}\right) = 8670 \text{ mg}$$

- More than one tool may be needed to complete the conversion. For example: How many inches are there in 3.5 m?

$$3.5 \text{ m} \left(\frac{100 \text{ cm}}{\text{m}}\right)\left(\frac{1 \text{ in}}{2.54 \text{ cm}}\right) = 137.8 \text{ in}$$

Using the Tools in the RP Method

- Write a ratio with x followed by the units of the answer on top and the given on the bottom. Using the 8.67 g to mg example above:

$$\frac{x \text{ mg}}{8.67 \text{ g}}$$

- Find a ratio in the tool shed with mg on top and g on the bottom. This is the reference ratio which will be compared to the ratio containing the unknow. Place an equal sign between them.

$$\frac{x \text{ mg}}{8.67 \text{ g}} = \frac{1000 \text{ mg}}{1 \text{ g}}$$

- **Solve for x mg. (8.67 g)(1000 mg) then divide by 1 g. x mg = 8670 mg**
- If more than one tool is needed, set up another problem with the first answer as your given, or preferably, use the DA method.

Unit Conversion Exercise using Dimensional Analysis

Given to be Converted	Conversion Factor (Tool)	Units of the Answer	Answer: (Given)(Tool)
3.5 g	1000 mg/g	mg	3500 mg
3400 g	1 kg/1000 g	kg	3.4 kg
25 mg		g	
8.1 kg		lb	
320 mg		g	
3 tbs		tsp	
245 cm		m	
2.2 kg		lb	
967 mcg		mg	
45 mg		mcg	
188 lb		kg	
2.5 L		mL	
502 g		kg	
89 mm		cm	
400 mL		L	
923 g		kg	
8 kg		g	
389 mL		L	
25 mm		cm	

Dosage Calculations for Nursing Students

Given to be Converted	Conversion Factor (Tool)	Units of the Answer	Answer: (Given)(Tool)
9.5 in		cm	
50 g		mg	
0.25 L		mL	
45 cm		in	
679 cm		m	
90 g		kg	
245 lb		kg	

Unit Conversion Exercise using Ratio Proportion

Given	Units of the Answer	Set up Equation	Answer (Solve for x)
3.5 g	mg	$\dfrac{x\ mg}{3.5\ g} = \dfrac{1000\ mg}{1\ g}$	**3500 mg**
3400 g	kg	$\dfrac{x\ kg}{3400\ g} = \dfrac{1\ kg}{1000\ g}$	**3.4 kg**
25 mg	g		
8.1 kg	lb		
320 mg	g		
3 tbs	tsp		
245 cm	m		
2.2 kg	lb		
967 mcg	mg		

Dosage Calculations for Nursing Students

Given	Units of the Answer	Set up Equation	Answer (Solve for x)
45 mg	mcg		
188 lb	kg		
2.5 L	mL		
502 g	kg		
89 mm	cm		
400 mL	L		
923 g	kg		
8 kg	g		
3.2 m	cm		
389 mL	L		
25 mm	cm		
9.5 in	cm		
50 g	mg		
0.25 L	mL		
45 cm	in		
679 cm	m		
90 g	kg		
245 lb	kg		

Chapter 9
Dosage Calculations

Terminology:

- **Dose:** The quantity of drug administered at a single time.
- **Dosage:** The dose information along with other pertinent information relating to the frequency, duration, route of administration, etc. of the dose.
  - Example: A patient is prescribed 500 mg orally three times daily for 10 days. The dose is 500 mg; the dosage is 500 mg orally three times daily for 10 days.
- **mg/kg/day:** Amount of drug in mg administered per kg of body weight each day.
  - **mg/(kg·day)** is mathematically equivalent and easier to use in calculations.

Step 1) Read the problem thoroughly looking for these three components:

- **The Units of the Answer:** The problem may say something like: How many mL, tablets, mg, teaspoonfuls, etc. will the patient take? Or it may say something less specific, like: What is the weight of, the volume of, how much suspension will be needed?
- **The Given of the Problem:** The problem may say something like, "A prescription is written for 10 mg, 20 mL, 1 g, etc.." or it may say, "A patient is to receive 250 mg, 5 mL, etc."
- **One or More Ratios:** All problems (other than simple unit conversions) will have a ratio somewhere in the problem; you just must learn to recognize it. It may be something like: 250 mg per 5 mL, a 50 mg tablet, 400 mcg per mL, 3 g in 100 mL. "Off the shelf" ratios may be required to complete the calculation.

Step 2) All the following problems can be solved using DA with the following equation:

- (Given)(Ratio 1)(Ratios 2, 3,...if needed) = Answer

Once the three components have been identified, the problem can be set up and solved.

Example: A patient is to receive a dose of 500 mg of amoxicillin. The pharmacy has a bottle of amoxicillin 250 mg per 5mL suspension. How many mL of the suspension will the patient receive each dose?

- Units of the answer: mL
- The given: 500mg
- The ratio: $\left(\dfrac{250 \text{ mg}}{5 \text{ mL}}\right)$

Step 3) The problem can now be set up:

- Write down the given and the units of the answer with an equal sign in between.

$$500 \text{ mg} = \text{mL}$$

- The ratio is the tool which will be used to change the units of the given (mg) into the units of the answer (mL). Remember, the ratios always equal 1 and can be flipped upside down if needed. The ratio must be placed so the units of the given are canceled out, leaving only the units of the answer. In this case, the ratio must be flipped putting mL on top and mg on the bottom.

$$500 \text{ mg} \left(\frac{5 \text{ mL}}{250 \text{ mg}}\right) = 10 \text{ mL}$$

Dosage Exercise Set 1

1) A patient has an order for 400 mg of a medication which is available as 500 mg/3 mL. How many mL will be administered?

2) The doctor has ordered a dose of 800 mg. The medication is available as 200 mg/10 mL. How many milliliters will need to be drawn up to fill the order?

3) A patient has an order for 1500 mcg. You have 500 mcg tablets available. How many tablets will be needed to fill the order?

4) The doctor has ordered 800 mg of a drug which is available in 10 mL vials of 100 mg/mL. How many mL will be administered?

5) A patient has an order for 14,000 units of heparin. It is available as 10,000 units/mL in a 10 mL vial. How many milliliters are needed?

6) The doctor has ordered a dose of 65 mg. The medication is available as 100 mg/10 mL. How many milliliters will need to be drawn up to fill the order?

7) How many mcg of levothyroxine are contained in 2 tablets of levothyroxine 0.125 mg?

8) A patient has an order for 1.6 mg. You have 0.4 mg tablets available. How many tablets will be needed to fill the order?

9) You will be administrating 5 mL of a drug which has a strength of 25 mg/mL. How many mg will be administered?

10) A prescriber has ordered 375 mg of a drug which comes in a strength of 75 mg/mL. How many mL will be administered?

Dosage Exercise Set 2

1) A patient is to receive 150 mg of a drug per day divided into 3 equal doses. The drug is available in 10 mL vials of 10 mg/mL. How many mL will be administered for each dose?

2) A patient who weighs 185 lb is to receive a dosage of 2 mg/kg/day for 4 days. The drug is available in 10 mL vials of 50 mg/mL. How many total mL will be administered over the 4 days.

3) A patient is ordered 600 mg/day in 4 equal doses. The drug is available in 10 mL vials of 50 mg/mL. How many mL will the patient receive in 1 dose?

4) A patient is prescribed 250 mg 3 times daily for 10 days. The drug is available in 125 mg capsules. How many capsules will be administered per dose?

5) An 80 kg patient is prescribed 3 mg/kg/day for 7 days. The drug is available in 5 mL vials of 50 mg/mL. How many vials will be needed for the 7 days? Tip: Convert 3 mg/kg/day to 3 mg/(kg*day).

6) A patient is to receive 5 mL of a drug 3 times daily for 10 days. The drug is available in a strength of 25 mg/mL in a bottle of 240 mL. How many mg will the patient receive in each dose?

7) A patient weighs 205 lbs and is prescribed a dosage of 600 mg IV given over 2 hours. The drug is available in 10 mL vials of 100 mg/ mL. How many mL will be administered?

8) A patient is to receive a dosage of 34 mg/kg/day each day for 60 days. The patient weighs 196 lb. The drug is available in 20 mL vials of 200 mg/mL. How many vials will be required for the 60 day course of therapy?

9) A patient is prescribed 250 mg 4 times daily. The drug is available in 125 mg capsules. How many capsules will be administered each day?

10) Order: 25 mcg/kg/day divided into 4 equal doses. The patient's weight is 176 lb. The drug is available in 10 mL vials of 250 mcg/mL. How many mL will be administered for each dose?

Chapter 10
IV Flow Rate Calculations

Terminology:

- **IV:** Abbreviation for intravenous, meaning administered into a vein.
- **drop factor:** The number of drops (gtts) per mL. Macrodrip tubing comes 10, 15, 20 gtts/mL while microdrip tubing is 60 gtt/mL.
- **VTBI:** Volume to be infused.
- **flow rate/infusion rate/drip rate:** The volume of solution or weight of drug delivered over time. The units are usually gtts/min, mL/hour or mg/hour.

These problems are solved in the same manner as unit conversion and dosage problems. There is a given, units of the answer, and one or more ratios which will be used to convert the units of the given into the units of the answer.

The general setup of an IV flow rate problem is:

$$(Given)(Ratios) = Answer$$

The problem will supply you with the given and the units of the answer. The ratios will either be supplied in the problem, or you may have to use your own (60 min/h, 1000 mcg/mg, etc.).

There are three types of IV Flow rate problems:

- The **rate to rate** problem is the most common. For example: An IV is running at a rate of 1 Liter per hour with a drop factor of 20 (20 drops/mL). What is the rate in drops/min?
  If the units of the answer are a rate, the given must be a rate.

(Rate)(Ratios) = Rate

- The **time to quantity** problem will give you a time duration and ask for the quantity of something (mL, mg, mg/kg, mEq) delivered over that duration. For example: An IV with a flow rate of 500 mL/h has been running for 2 hours. What volume of fluid has been administered?
  If the units of the answer are a quantity, the given must be a time duration.

(Time)(Ratios) = Quantity

- The **quantity to time** is just the opposite of the time to quantity problem. You will be given a quantity of something and asked for the time duration to administer it. For example: How long will it take to administer 1 L of fluid at the rate of 250 mL/h?
  If the units of the answer are a time duration, the given must be a quantity.

Dosage Calculations for Nursing Students

(Quantity)(Ratios) = Time

Examples:

1) 1000 mL is infused over 4 hours using an infusion set with a drop factor of 10 (10 gtts/mL). Calculate the flow rate in gtts/min.

Step 1) Look at the units of the answer. Gtts/min is a rate, so the given must be a rate. The only other rate in the problem is 1000 mL/4 h. Write these down with an equal sign.

$$\frac{1000 \text{ mL}}{4 \text{ h}} = \frac{\text{gtts}}{\text{min}}$$

Now you can see that you have to change mL to gtts and h to min. The ratio of $\frac{10 \text{ gtts}}{\text{mL}}$ will change mL to gtts and the ratio $\frac{1 \text{ h}}{60 \text{ min}}$ will change hours to minutes.

Step 2) Arrange the ratios so the unwanted units cancel leaving the units of the answer.

$$\frac{1000 \text{ mL}}{4 \text{ h}} \left(\frac{10 \text{ gtts}}{\text{mL}}\right) \left(\frac{1 \text{ h}}{60 \text{ min}}\right) = \frac{\text{gtts}}{\text{min}}$$

Step 3) Take out your calculator and do the calculations. Multiply everything on top and divide by everything on the bottom, giving the answer of 41.7 gtts/min which is rounded to 42 gtts/min.

$$\frac{1000 \text{ mL}}{4 \text{ h}} \left(\frac{10 \text{ gtts}}{\text{mL}}\right) \left(\frac{1 \text{ h}}{60 \text{ min}}\right) = 42 \frac{\text{gtts}}{\text{min}}$$

2) A patient has an order for regular insulin at the rate of 18 units/hour. The solution is 100 mL with 100 units of regular insulin. An infusion set with a drop factor of 20 is being used. What will be the flow rate in gtts/min?

Step 1) Looking at the units of the answer you see gtts/min, so you know the given must be a rate. The only other rate in the problem is 18 units/hour, so you know this is the given.

$$\frac{18 \text{ units}}{\text{h}} = \frac{\text{gtts}}{\text{min}}$$

You will have to change units to gtts and hours to minutes. It will take two ratios to change units to gtts, $\frac{100 \text{ mL}}{100 \text{ units}}$ and $\frac{20 \text{ gtts}}{\text{mL}}$. The ratio of $\frac{1 \text{ h}}{60 \text{ min}}$ will change hours to minutes.

Step 2) Arrange the ratios so the unwanted units cancel leaving the units of the answer. Double check everything and do the calculations.

$$\frac{18 \text{ units}}{\text{h}} \left(\frac{100 \text{ mL}}{100 \text{ units}}\right) \left(\frac{20 \text{ gtts}}{\text{mL}}\right) \left(\frac{1 \text{ h}}{60 \text{ min}}\right) = 6 \frac{\text{gtts}}{\text{min}}$$

Dosage Calculations for Nursing Students

3) A patient has an order for a drug to be infused at the rate of 25 mg/kg/h. A 1 L bag contains 10 g of the drug and the patient weighs 80 kg. An infusion set with a drop factor of 15 is being used. What is the flow rate in gtts/min?

This problem looks a little different because it contains the rate 25 mg/kg/h. This means (25 mg/kg)/h. You can either enter the rate as $\frac{25 \text{ mg/kg}}{h}$ or my prefered way $\frac{25 \text{ mg}}{\text{kg h}}$, which is mathematically equivalent.

Step 1) Look at the units of the answer. Gtts/min is a rate, so the given must be a rate. The only other rate in the problem is 25 mg/kg/h. Write these down with an equal sign.

$$\frac{25 \text{ mg}}{\text{kg h}} = \frac{\text{gtts}}{\text{min}}$$

You will have to change mg to gtt and h to minutes. kg is not changed to anything, but rather eliminated from the equation. The patient's weight is part of the given and will be inserted above the line to eliminate kg.

Step 2) Arrange the ratios and the patient's weight so the unwanted units cancel leaving the units of the answer. Double check everything and do the calculations.

$$\frac{25 \cancel{\text{mg}}}{\cancel{\text{kg}} \text{ h}} \left(\frac{80 \cancel{\text{kg}}}{1}\right) \left(\frac{1 \cancel{\text{L}}}{10 \cancel{\text{g}}}\right) \left(\frac{1 \cancel{\text{g}}}{1000 \cancel{\text{mg}}}\right) \left(\frac{1000 \cancel{\text{mL}}}{\cancel{\text{L}}}\right) \left(\frac{15 \text{ gtts}}{\cancel{\text{mL}}}\right) \left(\frac{1 \cancel{\text{h}}}{60 \text{ min}}\right) = 50 \frac{\text{gtts}}{\text{min}}$$

4) Calculate the length of time required to infuse a 1000 mL bag at the rate of 50 mL/h.

Step 1) Look at the units of the answer. Although it doesn't say "Calculate the number of hours", you can figure that out yourself. Since the units of the answer is a time duration, you know that the given must be a quantity. The only quantity in the problem is 1000 mL.

$$1000 \text{ mL} = \text{hours}$$

Step 2) Whenever you have a time to quantity or quantity to time problem, one of the ratios must be a rate. The only rate in the problem is 50 mL/h, so you know that must be part of the equation.

$$1000 \cancel{\text{mL}} \left(\frac{1 \text{ h}}{50 \cancel{\text{mL}}}\right) = 20 \text{ h}$$

5) An IV has been running for 2 hours at the rate of 40 mL/h. How many mL have been administered?

This is an example of a simple time to quantity problem. The units of the answer are mL, so the given must be a time duration.

$$2\,\text{h} \quad = \quad \text{mL}$$

The rate of 40 mL/h will change h to mL.

$$2\,\cancel{\text{h}}\left(\frac{40\text{ mL}}{\cancel{\text{h}}}\right) = 80\text{ mL}$$

Summary

1) Look at the units of the answer.

- If it is a rate, the given will be a rate.
- If it is a duration of time, the given will be a quantity.
- If it is a quantity, the given will be a duration of time.

2) Compare the given to the units of the answer.

3) Insert the ratios so the unwanted units cancel leaving the units of the answer.

4) Double check everything and do the calculations.

IV Flow Rate Exercise

Calculate the flow rate in mL/h.

1) 1000 mL infused over 5 h.

2) 250 mL infused over 2 h.

Calculate the flow rate in gtts/min. Round to the nearest drop.

3) 1000 mL infused over 4 hours using an infusion set with a drop factor of 10 (10 gtts/mL).

4) 250 mL infused over 2 hours using an infusion set with a drop factor of 15.

5) 2 L infused over 24 hours using an infusion set with a drop factor of 20.

6) 100 mL infused over 1 hour using an infusion set with a drop factor of 10.

7) 1000 mL infused over 5 hours using an infusion set with a drop factor of 20.

Dosage Calculations for Nursing Students

Calculate the length of time required to infuse the following volumes.

8) A 1000 mL bag infused at the rate of 45 mL/h.

9) A 1000 mL bag infused at the rate of 45 mL/h using an infusion set with a drop factor of 20.

10) A 1000 mL bag infused at the rate of 45 mL/h using an infusion set with a drop factor of 10.

11) A 1 L bag infused at the rate of 50 gtts/min using an infusion set with a drop factor of 15.

12) A 500 mL bag infused at the rate of 25 gtts/min using an infusion set with a drop factor of 20.

Answer the following. Round to the nearest drop or mL.

13) A patient has an order for regular insulin at the rate of 18 units/hour. The solution is 100 mL with 100 units of regular insulin. An infusion set with a drop factor of 20 is being used. What will be the flow rate in gtts/min? What is the flow rate in mL/h?

14) A patient has an order for a drug to be infused at the rate of 5 mcg/kg/min. A 500 mL bag contains 250 mg of the drug and the patient weighs 185 pounds. An infusion set with a drop factor of 20 is being used. What is the flow rate in gtts/min? What is the flow rate in mL/h?

15) A patient has an order for a drug to be infused at the rate of 25 mg/kg/h. A 1 L bag contains 10 g of the drug and the patient weighs 80 kg. An infusion set with a drop factor of 15 is being used. What is the flow rate in gtts/min? What is the flow rate in mL/h?

Chapter 11
Percent, Percent Strength, Ratio Strength

Percent

The three key concepts in understanding percent are:

- **Percent means per 100.** 50% is 50 parts per 100, or $\frac{50}{100}$.

- **100% equals 1.** Since 100% = 1, the corresponding conversion factors are $\left(\frac{100\%}{1}\right)$ and $\left(\frac{1}{100\%}\right)$, which is the same as multiplying or dividing by 100%.

- **The percent sign (%) will cancel itself out just as the units of measurement cancel themselves out.** $\frac{12\%}{100\%} = \frac{12}{100}$

Converting a Number to a Percent

- **Convert a number to a percent by multiplying by 100%.**
- **Example: Convert 0.30 to a percent.** 0.30 (100%) = 30%.
  - ➢ 100% = 1, so the value of 0.30 has not changed, only the appearance.

Converting a Percent to a Number

- **Convert a percent to a number by dividing by 100%. If you wish, you can multiply by $\left(\frac{1}{100\%}\right)$, which is the same thing.**
- **Example: Convert 35% to a number.**

$$\left(\frac{35\%}{100\%}\right) = 0.35.$$

Converting a Fraction to a Percent

- **Convert a fraction to a percent by multiplying the fraction by 100%.**
- **Example: Convert 1/4 to a percent.** 1/4 (100%)= 25%

Summing up: To add the % sign, multiply by 100%. To remove the % sign, divide by 100%. (Yes, you multiply or divide by 100%, NOT 100.)

More Examples

Convert the following numbers to percent.

Number	Percent
0.87	0.87 (100%) = 87%
1.67	1.67 (100%) = 167%
0.0056	0.0056 (100%) = 0.56%
0.36	0.36 (100%) = 36%
3	3 (100%) = 300%
1.1	1.1 (100%) = 110%
0.9944	0.9944 (100%) = 99.44%

Convert the following percents to numbers.

Percent	Number
89%	89%/100% = 0.89
0.25%	0.25%/100% = 0.0025
157%	157%/100% = 1.57
99.44%	99.44%/100% = 0.9944
56.1%	56.1%/100% = 0.561
25%	25%/100% = 0.25
34%	34%/100% = 0.34

Convert the following fractions to percents.

Fraction	Percent
5/6	5/6 (100%) = 83.3%
9/10	9/10 (100%) = 90%
2/20	2/20 (100%) = 10%
1/4	1/4 (100%) = 25%
34/50	34/50 (100%) = 68%
2/8	2/8 (100%) = 25%
13/99	13/99 (100%) = 13.1%

Dosage Calculations for Nursing Students

Percent Exercise

1) Convert the following numbers to percents using the format in the examples below.

0.35	(0.35)(100%)=35%
15/17	(15/17)(100%)=88.24%
0.98	
1.78	
3.99	
0.05	
0.003	
1.25	
6/9	
5.45	
9.95	
0.005	

2) Convert the following percents to numbers using the format in the example below.

56%	$\dfrac{56\%}{100\%} = 0.56$
3.5%	
99%	
101%	
34.5%	
85.67%	
3.35%	
3%	

Calculating Percent Change

Occasionally you will be required to calculate the percent change between two quantities.

Example 1) A patient's weight increased from 81 kg to 84 kg. What is the percent change?

- The formula to calculate percent change is:

$$\frac{\text{Final} - \text{Initial}}{\text{Initial}} (100\%) = \%\ \text{Change}$$

- The patient's final weight is 84 kg.
- The patient's initial weight is 81 kg.

$$\frac{84\ \text{kg} - 81\ \text{kg}}{81\ \text{kg}} (100\%) = \frac{3\ \text{kg}}{81\ \text{kg}} (100\%) = 3.7\%$$

Example 2) A patient is prescribed 2.5 mg of a drug and the prescriber increased to dose to 3 mg. What is the percent change?

$$\frac{3\ \text{mg} - 2.5\ \text{mg}}{2.5\ \text{mg}} (100\%) = \frac{0.5\ \text{mg}}{2.5\ \text{mg}} (100\%) = 20\%$$

Percent Change Exercise

For the following calculate the percent change and indicate if it is an increase or decrease.

1) A patient's weight is 171 lb. on Monday and 173 lb. on Thursday.

2) A patient weighs 192 lb. on Wednesday and one week later weighs 85 kg.

3) A drug is dosed at 5 mcg/kg/min then increased to 6.2 mcg/kg/min.

4) You got a merit raise in pay from $48.75 per hour to $50.00 per hour.

Percent Strength

The only difference between percent strength and percent is that percent strength includes units of weight and volume.

- **Weight, in a percent strength, is always expressed in units of gram (g).**
- **Volume, in a percent strength, is always expressed in units of milliliter (mL).**

The Four Types of Mixtures, also Called Solutions

Weight in Weight $\left(\frac{w}{w}\right)$: An example is 1 g of hydrocortisone (the solute) in 100 g of final cream (the solution). This is a 1% hydrocortisone cream.

Weight in Volume $\left(\frac{w}{v}\right)$: An example is 1 g of NaCl (the solute) in 100 mL of NaCl solution (the solution). This is a 1% NaCl solution.

Volume in Volume $\left(\frac{v}{v}\right)$: An example is 1 mL of ethanol (the solute) in 100 mL of final product (the solution) (1 mL ethanol mixed with 99 mL of water). This is a 1% ethanol solution.

Volume in weight $\left(\frac{v}{w}\right)$: This type of solution is not very common. An example is 10 mL of glycerin in 100 g glycerin ointment. This is a 10% glycerin ointment.

A 1% NaCl solution is 1% $\frac{w}{v}$ NaCl solution. Sometimes the units $\frac{w}{w}, \frac{w}{v}, \frac{v}{v}, \frac{v}{w}$ are not included in the problem and must be added. If it is weighed, it is w, if the volume is measured, it is v. Note that occasionally liquids are expressed in weight.

The Key to Solving these Problems

- **Substitute g for w and mL for v in the ratios and units of the answer.**
- **Preform the calculations.**
- **Substitute w and v back in the final answer, if required.**

Example: How many grams of NaCl are in 45 mL of 2% $\frac{w}{v}$ NaCl solution?

- This problem can be completed in one step. Substitute g for w and mL for v, multiply by 45 mL and divide by 100%.

$$45 \text{ mL} \left(\frac{2\% \text{ g}}{100\% \text{ mL}}\right) = 0.9 \text{ g}$$

See how nicely mL and % cancel out? If the problem asked for the number of mg, add the conversion factor $\left(\frac{1000 \text{ mg}}{\text{g}}\right)$.

$$45 \text{ mL} \left(\frac{2\% \text{ g}}{100\% \text{ mL}}\right) \left(\frac{1000 \text{ mg}}{\text{g}}\right) = 900 \text{ mg}$$

Calculate the Percent Strength from Weight and Volume

Calculate the percent strength of a solution by setting up the problem with the given and the units of the answer. The final units of the answer will be % w/v, % w/w, % v/v, or % v/w, but substitute g and mL for w and v.

Example: What is the percent strength of a solution if there are 985 mg of NaCl in 2.5 L?

- Write down the given and the units of the answer:

$$\frac{985 \text{ mg}}{2.5 \text{ L}} = \quad \% \; \frac{g}{mL}$$

It is now easy to see that mg must be converted to g, L converted to mL, and the % must be added.

- Convert mg to g by multiplying by $\left(\frac{1 \text{ g}}{1000 \text{ mg}}\right)$
- Convert L to mL by multiplying by $\left(\frac{1 \text{ L}}{1000 \text{ mL}}\right)$.
- Add the % sign by multiplying by 100%.

$$\frac{985 \text{ mg}}{2.5 \text{ L}} \left(\frac{1 \text{ g}}{1000 \text{ mg}}\right)\left(\frac{1 \text{ L}}{1000 \text{ mL}}\right) 100\% = 0.0394\% \; \frac{g}{mL}$$

- Substitute w for g and v for mL in the final answer: $0.0394\% \; \frac{w}{v}$

Percent Strength Exercise

Express the following as percent strength solution and include the type of solution (w/w, w/v, v/v, v/w).

1) 7 g KCl in 200 mL

2) 3.5 g NaCl in 1000 mL

3) 7.9 mg NaHCO$_3$ in 100 mL

4) 5 mcg NaCl in 0.25 mL

5) 45 g NaCl in 3 L

6) 3 g HC in 200 g HC ointment

Dosage Calculations for Nursing Students

7) 5 g coal tar in 300 g coal tar ointment

8) 5 mg betamethasone in 10 g betamethasone ointment

9) 20 g urea in 40 g urea ointment

10) 18 g salicylic acid in 300 g salicylic acid cream

11) 900 mL IPA in 1000 mL IPA solution

12) 40 mL ETOH in 100 mL ETOH solution

Answer the following:

13) How many mg of NaCl are in 10 mL of 0.9% NaCl (normal saline)?

14) How many g of NaCl are in 2 L of NS (normal saline)?

15) How many g of KCl are in 473 mL of 20% KCl?

16) How many mg of bupivacaine are in 30 mL of 0.5% bupivacaine solution?

17) How many mg of lidocaine are in 100 mL of 1% lidocaine?

18) How many mcg of NaCl are in 1 drop of 0.9% NaCl if there are 20 drops/mL?

19) How many mL of ETOH are in 60 mL of 80 proof (40% ETOH) tequila?

20) How many g of HC are in 500 g of 2.5% HC ointment?

Ratio Strength

- Very occasionally, drug strengths are expressed as ratio strengths.
- These calculations have similarities to percent strength calculations.
  - The units are always g and mL.
  - Solutions may be w/w, w/v, v/v, or v/w.
- **The conventional format is 1:another number, where the other number is the amount of final product. Examples: 1:100, 1:500, 1:10,000.**
  - A 1:100 w/w preparation is 1 g active ingredient in 100 g of final product. It is not 1 g of active ingredient mixed with 100 g of inactive ingredient.
  - A 1:100 w/v solution is 1 g active ingredient in 100 mL solution.
  - A 1:100 v/v solution is 1 mL of active ingredient in 100 mL solution.
  - A 1:100 v/w solution is 1 mL of active ingredient in 100 g of product.
- Keys to preforming calculations involving ratio strengths.
  - Determine the type of solution (w/w, w/v, v/v, v/w).
  - Assign the units of g to w and mL to v.
  - Convert from the colon format into the fraction format with the units attached. Example: 1:1000 w/v becomes 1 g/1000 mL.
  - Proceed with calculations using DA or RP.

Example: How many mg of epinephrine are in 45 mL of a 1:10,000 solution of epinephrine?

- This is a **w** (mg) of epinephrine in **v** (45 mL) solution.
- 1:10,000 w/v is 1 g:10,000 mL
- 1 g:10,000 mL converted to fraction format is $\left(\frac{1 \text{ g}}{10,000 \text{ mL}}\right)$.
- Proceed with calculations using DA.

$$45 \text{ mL} \left(\frac{1 \text{ g}}{10,000 \text{ mL}}\right)\left(\frac{1000 \text{ mg}}{\text{g}}\right) = 4.5 \text{ mg}$$

Important: Many fatalities have resulted from incorrect calculations involving ratio strength, with epinephrine being one of the most common drugs involved. Be very careful when preforming ratio strength calculations. Most drugs labeled with ratio strength will include the strength listed in mg/mL, which is safer to use.

Ratio Strength Exercise

1) How many grams of active ingredient are in 500 mL of a 1:10,000 solution?

2) How many grams of active ingredient are in 40 mL of a 1:200 solution?

3) How many grams of active ingredient are in 600 g of a 1:25 w/w preparation?

4) How many mg of active ingredient are in 800 mL of a 1:10,000 solution?

5) How many mcg are in 10 mL of a 1:100,000 solution?

6) You have a 10 mL vial which is labeled 1:10,000 and are asked to draw up 0.4 mg of drug. How many mL would you draw?

7) You have a 50 mL vial which is labeled 1:1000 and are asked to draw up 1 mg. How many mL would you draw?

8) You have a solution which is 1:10,000 w/v. What is the percentage strength?

9) What is the percentage strength of a 1:100 w/v solution?

10) You have a 100 mL vial which is labeled 1:1000. How many mg are in 25 mL of the solution?

Chapter 12
Milliequivalent Calculations

As nurses, you will probably not be required to convert between mg and mEq, but some of you may want to go above and beyond what is required. If nothing else, learning the terminology and key concepts listed below will be helpful.

Terminology:
- **Electrolytes:** Ions which are important to the function of the body. (Na^+, K^+, Cl^-, etc.)
- **Ion**: An atom or group of atoms that has either lost or gained electrons and carries either a positive or negative charge.
- **Cation:** A positively charged ion (pronounced cat-ion).
- **Anion**: A negatively charged ion.
- **Valence:** The simple definition is the number of charges on the ion.
- **Atomic Mass/Atomic Weight**: For purposes of this book, these terms are used interchangeably. They are relative weights of the elements. For example, hydrogen has an atomic mass of 1 while carbon has an atomic mass of 12. An atom of carbon is twelve times as heavy as an atom of hydrogen. There are no units on atomic masses.

Key Concepts to Understanding Milliequivalent Calculations

- mEq calculations involve quantities of ions and charges, not weights. Think dozens of eggs, not pounds of coffee beans.
- A millimole (mmole) is 1/1000 of a mole (mol) or 6.022×10^{20} of anything.
- A mEq is a mmol of charges.
- Examples:
- 1 mmol of NaCl = 1 mmol of Na^+ and 1 mmol of Cl^-.
- Na^+ and Cl^- each have one charge.
- 1 mmol of NaCl = 1 mEq of Na^+ and 1 mEq Cl^-.
- 1 mmol of $MgSO_4$ = 1 mmol of Mg^{+2} and 1 mmol of SO_4^{-2}.
- Mg^{+2} and SO_4^{-2} each have two charges.
- 1 mmol of $MgSO_4$ = 2 mEq of Mg^{+2} and 2 mEq of SO_4^{-2}.

Converting Between mg and mEq

- The weight of a mmol of the electrolyte and the valence must be known.

- Determine the weight of a mmol of the electrolyte by looking up the atomic mass and adding mg to the end to give you the mg/mmol. For example, the atomic mass of potassium (K) is 39.1, which equates to 39.1 mg/mmol.
- Determine the valence by looking it up. The common electrolytes and their valences are listed in the milliequivalent exercise.

Example: How many mEq of KCl are in 300 mg of KCl?

- The formula mass (mass of K^+ + Cl^-) is 74.6, meaning 74.6 mg = 1 mmol. There is one charge on each ion, so 1 mmol = 1 mEq.

$$300 \text{ mg} \left(\frac{1 \text{ mmol}}{74.6 \text{ mg}}\right)\left(\frac{1 \text{ mEq}}{\text{mmol}}\right) = 4 \text{ mEq}$$

- It can also be stated that 4 mEq of KCl = 4 mEq of K^+ and 4 mEq of Cl^-.

Example: How many mEq of Mg^{+2} are in 300 mg of $MgSO_4$?

$$300 \text{ mg} \left(\frac{1 \text{ mmol}}{120.4 \text{ mg}}\right)\left(\frac{2 \text{ mEq}}{\text{mmol}}\right) = 5 \text{ mEq}$$

Milliequivalent Exercise

1) Look up the atomic masses (atomic weights) of the following elements. The atomic masses can be found on the periodic table or Google it. If you can't find them on your own, they are listed in the answers. Round to the nearest tenth.

Name	Atomic Symbol	Atomic Mass	Ionic Form
Hydrogen	H		H^+ (Hydrogen Ion)
Carbon	C		
Oxygen	O		
Sodium	Na		Na^+ (Sodium Ion)
Magnesium	Mg		Mg^{++} (Magnesium Ion)
Chlorine	Cl		Cl^- (Chloride Ion)
Potassium	K		K^+ (Potassium Ion)
Calcium	Ca		Ca^{++} (Calcium Ion)
Sulfur	S		

2) Now that you know the atomic masses of each of the elements, fill in the formula masses of the listed polyatomic ions (ions with more than one atom). Add up all the individual masses. CH_3COO^- has two carbon atoms, three hydrogen atoms, and two oxygen atoms.

Name	Chemical Formula	Formula Mass	Ionic Form
Acetate	CH_3COO^-		CH_3COO^-
Bicarbonate	HCO_3^-		HCO_3^-
Sulfate	SO_4^{-2}		SO_4^{-2}

3) Now that you know the above atomic and formula masses, you are ready to list the formula masses of the following ionic compounds.

Name	Chemical Formula	Formula Mass	Ionic Form
Sodium Chloride	NaCl		$Na^+ Cl^-$
Potassium Chloride	KCl		$K^+ Cl^-$
Calcium Chloride	$CaCl_2$		$Ca^{++} 2Cl^-$
Magnesium Chloride	$MgCl_2$		$Mg^{++} 2Cl^-$
Sodium Acetate	CH_3COONa		$Na^+ CH_3COO^-$
Potassium Acetate	CH_3COOK		$K^+ CH_3COO^-$
Magnesium Sulfate	$MgSO_4$		$Mg^{++} SO_4^{2-}$
Sodium Bicarbonate	$NaHCO_3$		$Na^+ HCO_3^-$

4) Fill in the table with the ratios of mg/mmol and mEq/mmol for each compound.

Name	Chemical Formula	mg/mmol (ratio)	mEq/mmol (ratio)
Sodium Chloride	NaCl		
Potassium Chloride	KCl		
Calcium Chloride	$CaCl_2$		
Magnesium Chloride	$MgCl_2$		
Sodium Acetate	CH_3COONa		
Potassium Acetate	CH_3COOK		
Magnesium Sulfate	$MgSO_4$		
Sodium Bicarbonate	$NaHCO_3$		

- You now have all the ratios needed to convert between mg and mEq.

Example: How many mEq are in 500 mg of $CaCl_2$?

- Calcium chloride has 111 mg per mmol and two mEq per mmol.
- These ratios can be written $\frac{111 \text{ mg}}{\text{mmol}}$ or $\frac{1 \text{ mmol}}{111 \text{ mg}}$ and $\frac{2 \text{ mEq}}{\text{mmol}}$ or $\frac{1 \text{ mol}}{2 \text{ mEq}}$.
- Set the problem up with the given and units of the answer.

$$500 \text{ mg} \qquad = \text{mEq}$$

- Insert the ratios in the usual way leaving only the units of the answer.

$$500 \text{ mg} \left(\frac{1 \text{ mmol}}{111 \text{ mg}}\right)\left(\frac{2 \text{ mEq}}{\text{mmol}}\right) = 9.0 \text{ mEq}$$

Answer the following.

5) How many mEq are contained in 746 mg of KCl?

6) How many mEq of calcium chloride are contained in 2 g of calcium chloride?

7) How many mEq of Ca^{++} are in 2 g of calcium chloride?

8) How many mg of magnesium sulfate are in 10 mEq of magnesium sulfate?

9) How many g of sodium acetate are in 12 mEq of sodium acetate?

10) How many mEq of NaCl are in 2 L of 0.9% NaCl?

11) How many mEq of KCl are in 30 mL of 10% KCl solution?

12) How many mEq of $MgSO_4$ are contained in 10 g of $MgSO_4$?

13) How many mg of Na^+ (just the sodium) are contained in 1.5 L of 10% NaCl?

14) Try this one if you wish. You have 2.5 L of 10% NaCl solution and your friend has 1.5 L of $MgSO_4$ solution. You have twice as many mEq of NaCl as your friend has of mEq of MgSO4. What is the percentage strength of your friend's $MgSO_4$?

Dosage Calculations for Nursing Students

Unit 4 Self-Assessment Exercise

Congratulations on finishing the book and starting the self-assessment exercise. This exercise is divided into two parts:

- Part 1: Basic calculations all nurses should be proficient in.
    - Unit Conversions
    - Rounding
    - Simple Roman Numeral Conversions
    - Military Time
    - Dosage Calculations
    - IV Flow Rate Calculations
    - Percent Conversions
    - Percent Change Calculations
    - Ratio Strength Calculations
    - Percent Strength Calculations
- Part 2: Calculations which you probably will not need in nursing but may be helpful in specialized nursing fields.
    - Unit conversions between lesser used metric units.
    - Scientific Notation Conversions
    - Milliequivalent Calculations

Please score yourself using the points assigned to each problem. Part 1 has a total of 79 points. Part 2 has a total of 16 points.

Part 1:

Convert the following (1 point each):

1) 1.1 L to mL

2) 3.2 cm to mm

3) 60 mcg to mg

4) 200 mcg to mg

5) 2.2 kg to lb.

6) 145 lb to kg

7) 30 mL to tsp

8) 130 mg to gr

9) 1 fl oz to tbs

10) 160 lb to kg

Round the following to the nearest tenth (1 point each):

Dosage Calculations for Nursing Students

11) 16.59 mg

12) 20.179 mg

13) 1.43 L

14) What is the Roman numeral for 5? (1 point)

15) What is the Roman numeral for 4? (1 point)

Convert the following times (1 point each):

16) 1:05 PM to military time.

17) 12:07 AM to military time.

18) 1430 to civilian time.

19-30: Calculate the amount to administer and round to the nearest tenth. 2 points each.

Order	150 mg IM
Available	300 mg/mL
Administer	

20)

Order	600 mg IV
Available	1 g/10 mL
Administer	

21)

Order	500 mg PO
Available	250 mg tab
Administer	

22)

Order	10 mg IV
Available	5 mg/mL
Administer	

23)

Order	2 mg/kg
Available	40 mg/mL
Pt Weight	62 kg
Administer	

24)

Order	5 mg/kg
Available	80 mg/mL
Pt Weight	190 lb
Administer	

25)

Order	1 mg/kg
Available	40 mg/mL
Pt Weight	176 lb
Administer	

26)

Order	5 mcg/kg
Available	30 mcg/mL
Pt Weight	12 kg
Administer	

27)

Order	8 mcg/kg
Available	100 mcg/mL
Pt Weight	126 lb
Administer	

28)

Order	6 mcg/kg/day divided into 4 equal doses.
Available	100 mcg/mL
Pt Weight	175 lb
Administer/dose	

29)

Order	2 mg/kg/day divided into 2 equal doses
Available	25 mg/mL
Pt Weight	120 lb
Administer/dose	

30)

Order	10 mg/kg/day divided into 3 equal doses
Available	20 mg/mL
Pt Weight	14 kg
Administer	

31-36: Calculate the following flow rates in mL/h. Round to the nearest mL. (2 points each)

31) Infuse 1500 mL over 6 hours.

32) Infuse 1000 mL over 4 hours 30 min.

33) Infuse 250 mL over 5 hours.

34-36: Calculate the following flow rates in gtts/min. (2 points each)

34) Infuse 500 mL over 6 hours with a drop factor of 20 (20 gtts/mL).

35) Infuse 1000 mL over 3 hours 15 min with a drop factor of 10.

36) Infuse 500 mL of 7 hours with a drop factor of 15.

37) You have an order to start a Pitocin infusion at 5 mUnits/min. You have on hand a 100 mL bag containing 10 Units of Pitocin. At what rate will you set the IV pump in mL/h? Round to the nearest mL/h. (3 points)

38) You have an order to start a DOPamine infusion at the rate of 4 mcg/kg/min on a 185 lb patient. You have a DOPamine 800 mg in 500 mL D5W. At what rate will you set the IV pump in mL/h? Round to the nearest tenth mL/h. (3 points)

39) You have an order to start a DOBUTtamine infusion at the rate of 2 mcg/kg/min on a 160 lb patient. You have on hand 500 mg DOBUTamine in 250 mL D5W. At what rate will you set the IV pump in mL/h? Round to the nearest tenth mL/h. (3 points)

40- 42: Convert each of the following decimal numbers into a percent. (1 point each)

40) 0.45

41) 0.02

42) 1.3

43-45: Convert the following percents into decimal numbers. (1 point each)

43) 67%

44) 32.1%

45) 101%

46) Your patient weighed 84 kg when admitted and now weighs 81 kg. What is the percent change to the nearest tenth of a percent? (2 points)

47) A patient's medication dosage went from 400 mg/day to 600 mg/day. What is the percent change to the nearest tenth of a percent? (2 points)

48) How many mcg of a drug are contained in 1 mL of a 1:10,000 solution? (2 points)

49) How many mg of NaCl are contained in 100 mL of 0.9% NaCl? (2 points)

50) A student is celebrating after finishing the dosage calculation class by drinking a margarita with 2 fl oz of 80 proof tequila in it. Proof is twice the percent v/v ethanol. How many mL of ethanol did she consume? (2 points)

End of Part 1, 79 total points possible. Calculate your percent score by dividing your total points by 79 then multiplying by 100%.

Part 2:

1-3: Convert the following (1 point each).

1) 302 ng to mg.

2) 2.5 dL to mL

3) 2.4 ML to L. (Note: ML is NOT the same as mL).

4-6: Write the following numbers in scientific notation (1 point each):

4) 0.000000682

5) 0.0000000002955

6) 1,590,000,000,000,000

7) T or F: A mEq of Na^+ weighs the same as a mEq of K^+. (1 point)

8) How many mEq of calcium chloride are contained in 1.6 g of calcium chloride? (3 points)

9) How many mEq of KCl are in 45 mL of 20% KCl solution? (3 points)

10) How many mg of sodium acetate are in 10 mEq of sodium acetate? (3 points)

End of part 2. 16 points possible.

Answers to Exercises

Rounding Exercise Answers				
	Round to the Nearest Tenth	Rounded Number		Round to the Nearest Hundredth	Rounded Number
1	6.88	6.9	26	89.568	89.57
2	7.54	7.5	27	45.789	45.79
3	2.22	2.2	28	1.005	1.01
4	3.98	4.0	28	2.895	2.90
5	78.53	78.5	30	3.997	4.00
6	99.23	99.2	31	7.894	7.89
7	101.16	101.2	32	3.433	3.43
8	5.44	5.4	33	2.222	2.22
9	99.99	100.0	34	1.111	1.11
10	53.247	53.2	35	8.895	8.90
11	9.355	9.4	36	3.578	3.58
12	100.01	100.0	37	2.2256	2.23
13	56.3756	56.4	38	90.3895	90.39
14	9.56	9.6	39	78.451	78.45
15	22.56	22.6	40	3.215	3.22
16	78.59	78.6	41	9.782	9.78
17	77.459	77.5	42	10.554	10.55
18	3.57	3.6	43	3.987	3.99
19	9.78	9.8	44	1.9954	2.00
20	23.598	23.6	45	2.493	2.49
21	78.3	78.3	46	8.523	8.52
22	78.303	73.3	47	9.672	9.67
23	798.32	798.3	48	4.956	4.96
24	8.06	8.1	49	2.225	2.23
25	9.11	9.1	50	3.987	3.99

Dosage Calculations for Nursing Students

Roman Numerals Exercise Answers

1) You must know the eight basic Roman numerals and their number counterparts: SS, I, V, X, L, C, D, M. Fill in the blanks on the following tables.

Roman Numeral	Number
SS	1/2
I	1
V	5
X	10
L	50
C	100
D	500
M	1000

Number	Roman Numeral
1/2	SS
1	I
5	V
10	X
50	L
100	C
500	D
1000	M

2) Fill in the blanks with the corresponding Roman numerals or numbers.

50	L			C	100		
100	C			5	V		
1/2	SS			10	X		
X	10			L	50		
M	1000			I	1		
5	V			X	10		
V	5			D	500		
500	D			M	1000		
L	50			X	10		
SS	1/2			V	5		
1000	M			L	50		
1	I			C	100		
D	500			5	V		
L	50			50	L		
M	1000			1000	M		
10	X			100	C		

3) Fill in the blanks with the corresponding Roman numerals.

1000	M	100	C	10	X	1	I
2000	MM	200	CC	20	XX	2	II
3000	MMM	300	CCC	30	XXX	3	III
		400	CD	40	XL	4	IV
		500	D	50	L	5	V

		600	DC	60	LX	6	VI
		700	DCC	70	LXX	7	VII
		800	DCCC	80	LXXX	8	VIII
		900	CM	90	XC	9	IX
						1/2	SS

4) Fill in the blanks with the appropriate number or Roman numeral.

10	X	LXX	70
30	XXX	20	XX
400	CD	CCC	300
DC	600	CD	400
2000	MM	CM	900
8	VIII	700	DCC
XC	90	50	L
40	XL	20	XX
60	LX	LXXX	80
200	CC	DCC	700
900	CM	600	DC
IV	4	CC	200
III	3	9	IX
SS	½ (0.5)	4	IV

5) Write the corresponding Roman numerals or numbers:

352   752

300	CCC	700	DCC
50	L	50	L
2	II	2	II
	CCCLII		**DCCLII**

3564   1437

3000	MMM	1000	M
500	D	400	CD
60	LX	30	XXX
4	IV	7	VII
	MMMDLXIV		**MCDXXXVII**

1369   3421

1000	M	3000	MMM
300	CCC	400	CD
60	LX	20	XX
9	IX	1	I
	MCCCLXIX		**MMMCDXXI**

MMDCLXVII

MM	2000
DC	600
LX	60
VII	7

2667

MCMLI

M	1000
CM	900
L	50
I	1

1951

CCCXLV

CCC	300
XL	40
V	5

345

DCLXII

DC	600
LX	60
II	2

662

Scientific Notation Exercise Answers

1) Convert the following numbers to scientific notation.

Number	Coefficient	# of Places from New Decimal Point to end of Original Number	Coefficient X 10 Raised to the Number of Places the Decimal Point was Moved
67,000	6.7	4	6.7×10^4
2,387,000	2.387	6	2.387×10^6
7,000,000	7	6	7×10^6
98,000	9.8	4	9.8×10^4
432,000,000	4.32	8	4.32×10^8
900,000,000	9	8	9×10^8
58,000,000,000	5.8	10	5.8×10^{10}
2,478,000,000	2.478	9	2.478×10^9
92,000,000	9.2	7	9.2×10^7
60,230,000,000	6.023	10	6.023×10^{10}
105,000	1.05	5	1.05×10^5

2) Convert the following decimal numbers to scientific notation.

Decimal Number	Coefficient	# of Places from New Decimal Point to Original Decimal Point	Coefficient X 10 Raised to the Negative Number of Places the Decimal Point was Moved
0.056	5.6	2	5.6×10^{-2}
0.000380	3.80	4	3.80×10^{-4}
0.00007	7	5	7×10^{-5}
0.00002039	2.039	5	2.039×10^{-5}
0.0005078	5.078	4	5.078×10^{-4}
0.00001832	1.832	5	1.832×10^{-5}
0.000650	6.50	4	6.50×10^{-4}
0.0000000012	1.2	9	1.2×10^{-9}
0.000054	5.4	5	5.4×10^{-5}
0.000783	7.83	4	7.83×10^{-4}
0.00034	3.4	4	3.4×10^{-4}

3) Convert the following numbers from scientific notation to numbers.

Scientific Notation	Coefficient	Exponent	# of Places to Move the Decimal Point to the Right	Number
5.62×10^6	5.62	6	6	5,620,000
7.8×10^7	7.8	7	7	78,000,000
9×10^5	9	5	5	900,000
6.02×10^7	6.02	7	7	60,200,000
1.05×10^4	1.05	4	4	10,500
9.78×10^9	9.78	9	9	9,780,000,000
6.99×10^3	6.99	3	3	6,990
3.78×10^8	3.78	8	8	378,000,000
4.0×10^8	4.0	8	8	400,000,000
7.66×10^5	7.66	5	5	766,000

4) Convert the following decimal numbers from scientific notation to decimal numbers.

Scientific Notation	Coefficient	Exponent	# of Places to Move the Decimal Point to the Left	Decimal Number
6.05×10^{-4}	6.05	-4	4	0.000605
2.3×10^{-7}	2.3	-7	7	0.00000023
7.80×10^{-4}	7.80	-4	4	0.000780
3.5×10^{-6}	3.5	-6	6	0.0000035
8.995×10^{-5}	8.995	-5	5	0.00008995
1.023×10^{-9}	1.023	-9	9	0.000000001023
5.00×10^{-4}	5.00	-4	4	0.000500
8.43×10^{-6}	8.43	-6	6	0.00000843
2.22×10^{-3}	2.22	-3	3	0.00222
1.6×10^{-7}	1.6	-7	7	0.00000016

Military Time Exercise Answers

Convert the following civilian times to military time.

1) 5:15 AM   **0515**

2) 12:25 AM   **0025**

3) 8:27 PM   **2027**

4) 11:19 PM   **2319**

5) 6:00 AM   **0600**

Convert the following military times to civilian times.

6) 0520   **5:20 AM**

7) 2301   **11:01 PM**

8) 1205   **12:05 PM**

9) 0610   **6:10 AM**

Dosage Calculations for Nursing Students

10) 1301   **1:01 PM**

11) You started work at 0600 and you ended work at 1400. You didn't get any lunch or breaks (poor you). How many hours did you work? **8 hours**

12) An IV was started at 1100 and ended at 2:30 PM. How many hours did it run?

   3.5 hours

13) You have the weekend off. You started watching your favorite Netflix series at 0730 on Saturday morning and finished at 0130 on Sunday. How many hours did you sit on the couch watching TV? **18 hours**

14) A patient is admitted at 0600 and pushes his call button 8 times between 0600 and 0616. What is the average time interval between button pushes? **2 minutes**

Unit Conversion Exercise using Dimensional Analysis Answers

Given to be Converted	Conversion Factor (Tool)	Units of the Answer	Answer: (Given)(Tool)
3.5 g	1000 mg/g	mg	3500 mg
3400 g	1 kg/1000 g	kg	3.4 kg
25 mg	1 g/1000 mg	g	0.025 g
8.1 kg	2.2 lb/kg	lb	17.8 lb
320 mg	1 g/1000 mg	g	0.320 g
3 tbs	3 tsp/tbs	tsp	9 tsp
245 cm	1 m/100 cm	m	2.45 m
2.2 kg	2.2 lb/kg	lb	4.8 lb
967 mcg	1 mg/1000 mcg	mg	0.967 mg
45 mg	1000 mcg/mg	mcg	45,000 mcg
188 lb	1 kg/2.2 lb	kg	85.5 kg
2.5 L	1000 mL/L	mL	2500 mL
502 g	1 kg/1000 g	kg	0.502 kg
89 mm	1 cm/10 mm	cm	8.9 cm
400 mL	1 L/1000 mL	L	0.400 L
923 g	1 kg/1000 g	kg	0.923 kg
8 kg	1000 g/kg	g	8000 g
3.2 m	100 cm/m	cm	320 cm
389 mL	1 L/1000 mL	L	0.389 L
25 mm	1 cm/10 mm	cm	2.5 cm
9.5 in	2.54 cm/in	cm	24.1 cm
50 g	1000 mg/g	mg	50,000 mg
0.25 L	1000 mL/L	mL	250 mL
45 cm	1 in/2.54 cm	in	17.7 in
679 cm	1 m/100 cm	m	6.79 m
90 g	1 kg/1000 g	kg	0.09 kg
245 lb	1 kg/2.2 lb	kg	111.4 kg

Unit Conversion Exercise using Ratio Proportion Answers

Given to be Converted	Units of the Answer	Set up Equation	Answer: Solve for x
3.5 g	mg	$\dfrac{x \text{ mg}}{3.5 \text{ g}} = \dfrac{1000 \text{ mg}}{1 \text{ g}}$	3500 mg

Dosage Calculations for Nursing Students

3400 g	kg	$\dfrac{x \text{ kg}}{3400 \text{ g}} = \dfrac{1 \text{ kg}}{1000 \text{ g}}$	3.4 kg
25 mg	g	$\dfrac{x \text{ g}}{25 \text{ mg}} = \dfrac{1 \text{ g}}{1000 \text{ mg}}$	0.025 g
8.1 kg	lb	$\dfrac{x \text{ lb}}{8.1 \text{ kg}} = \dfrac{2.2 \text{ lb}}{1 \text{ kg}}$	17.8 lb
320 mg	g	$\dfrac{x \text{ g}}{320 \text{ mg}} = \dfrac{1 \text{ g}}{1000 \text{ mg}}$	0.320 g
3 tbs	tsp	$\dfrac{x \text{ tsp}}{3 \text{ tbs}} = \dfrac{3 \text{ tsp}}{1 \text{ tbs}}$	9 tsp
245 cm	m	$\dfrac{x \text{ m}}{245 \text{ cm}} = \dfrac{1 \text{ m}}{100 \text{ cm}}$	2.45 m
2.2 kg	lb	$\dfrac{x \text{ lb}}{2.2 \text{ kg}} = \dfrac{2.2 \text{ lb}}{1 \text{ kg}}$	4.8 lb
967 mcg	mg	$\dfrac{x \text{ mg}}{967 \text{ mcg}} = \dfrac{1 \text{ mg}}{1000 \text{ mcg}}$	0.967 mg
45 mg	mcg	$\dfrac{x \text{ mcg}}{45 \text{ mg}} = \dfrac{1000 \text{ mcg}}{1 \text{ mg}}$	45,000 mcg
188 lb	kg	$\dfrac{x \text{ kg}}{188 \text{ lb}} = \dfrac{1 \text{ kg}}{2.2 \text{ lb}}$	85.5 kg
2.5 L	mL	$\dfrac{x \text{ mL}}{2.5 \text{ L}} = \dfrac{1000 \text{ mL}}{1 \text{ L}}$	2500 mL
502 g	kg	$\dfrac{x \text{ kg}}{502 \text{ g}} = \dfrac{1 \text{ kg}}{1000 \text{ g}}$	0.502 kg
89 mm	cm	$\dfrac{x \text{ cm}}{89 \text{ mm}} = \dfrac{1 \text{ cm}}{10 \text{ mm}}$	8.9 cm
400 mL	L	$\dfrac{x \text{ L}}{400 \text{ mL}} = \dfrac{1 \text{ L}}{1000 \text{ mL}}$	0.400 L
923 g	kg	$\dfrac{x \text{ kg}}{923 \text{ g}} = \dfrac{1 \text{ kg}}{1000 \text{ g}}$	0.923 kg
8 kg	g	$\dfrac{x \text{ g}}{8 \text{ kg}} = \dfrac{1000 \text{ g}}{1 \text{ kg}}$	8000 g
389 mL	L	$\dfrac{x \text{ L}}{389 \text{ mL}} = \dfrac{1 \text{ L}}{1000 \text{ mL}}$	0.389 L
25 mm	cm	$\dfrac{x \text{ cm}}{25 \text{ mm}} = \dfrac{1 \text{ cm}}{10 \text{ mm}}$	2.5 cm
9.5 in	cm	$\dfrac{x \text{ cm}}{9.5 \text{ in}} = \dfrac{2.54 \text{ cm}}{1 \text{ in}}$	24.1 cm
50 g	mg	$\dfrac{x \text{ mg}}{50 \text{ g}} = \dfrac{1000 \text{ mg}}{1 \text{ g}}$	50,000 mg

Dosage Calculations for Nursing Students

0.25 L	mL	$\dfrac{x\ mL}{0.25\ L} = \dfrac{1000\ mL}{1\ L}$	250 mL
45 cm	in	$\dfrac{x\ in}{45\ cm} = \dfrac{1\ in}{2.54\ cm}$	17.7 in
679 cm	m	$\dfrac{x\ m}{679\ cm} = \dfrac{1\ m}{100\ cm}$	6.79 m
90 g	kg	$\dfrac{x\ kg}{90\ g} = \dfrac{1\ kg}{1000\ g}$	0.09 kg
245 lb	kg	$\dfrac{x\ kg}{245\ lb} = \dfrac{1\ kg}{2.2\ lb}$	111.4 kg

Dosage Exercise Set 1 Answers

1) A patient has an order for 400 mg of a medication which is available as 500 mg/5 mL. How many mL will be administered?

Units of the answer	mL
Given	400 mg
Ratio(s) as stated	500 mg/5 ml
Ratios(s) as used	5 mL/500 mg

$$400\ mg \left(\dfrac{5\ mL}{500\ mg}\right) = 4\ mL$$

2) The doctor has ordered a dose of 800 mg. The medication is available as 200 mg/10 mL. How many milliliters will need to be drawn up to fill the order?

Units of the answer	mL
Given	800 mg
Ratio(s) as stated	200 mg/10 mL
Ratios(s) as used	10 mL/200 mg

$$800\ mg \left(\dfrac{10\ mL}{200\ mg}\right) = 40\ mL$$

3) A patient has an order for 1500 mcg. You have 500 mcg tablets available. How many tablets will be needed to fill the order?

Units of the answer	tablets
Given	1500 mcg
Ratio(s) as stated	500 mcg/tablet
Ratios(s) as used	1 tablet/500 mcg

$$1500\ mcg \left(\dfrac{1\ tablet}{500\ mcg}\right) = 3\ tablets$$

4) The doctor has ordered 800 mg of a drug which is available in 10 mL vials of 100 mg/mL. How many ml will be administered?

Dosage Calculations for Nursing Students

Units of the answer	mL
Given	800 mg
Ratio(s) as stated	100 mg/mL
Ratios(s) as used	1 mL/100 mg

$$800 \text{ mg} \left(\frac{1 \text{ mL}}{100 \text{ mg}}\right) = 8 \text{ mL}$$

5) A patient has an order for 14,000 units of heparin. It is available as 10,000 units/mL in a 10 mL vial. How many milliliters are needed?

Units of the answer	mL
Given	14,000 units
Ratio(s) as stated	10,000 units/mL 10 mL/vial
Ratios(s) as used	1 mL/10,000 units

$$14,000 \text{ units} \left(\frac{1 \text{ mL}}{10,000 \text{ units}}\right) = 1.4 \text{ mL}$$

6) The doctor has ordered a dose of 65 mg. The medication is available as 100 mg/10 mL. How many milliliters will need to be drawn up to fill the order?

Units of the answer	mL
Given	65 mg
Ratio(s) as stated	100 mg/10 mL
Ratios(s) as used	10 mL/100 mg

$$65 \text{ mg} \left(\frac{10 \text{ mL}}{100 \text{ mg}}\right) = 6.5 \text{ mL}$$

7) How many mcg of levothyroxine are contained in 2 tablets of levothyroxine 0.125 mg?

Units of the answer	mcg
Given	2 tablets
Ratio(s) as stated	0.125 mg/tab
Ratios(s) used	0.125 mg/tab 1000 mcg/mg

$$2 \text{ tablets} \left(\frac{0.125 \text{ mg}}{\text{tablet}}\right) \left(\frac{1000 \text{ mcg}}{\text{mg}}\right) = 250 \text{ mcg}$$

8) A patient has an order for 1.6 mg. You have 0.4 mg tablets available. How many tablets will be needed to fill the order?

Units of the answer	tablets
Given	1.6 mg
Ratio(s) as stated	0.4 mg/tablet

Ratios(s) as used	1 tablet/0.4 mg

$$1.6 \text{ mg} \left(\frac{1 \text{ tablet}}{0.4 \text{ mg}}\right) = 4 \text{ tablets}$$

9) You will be administrating 5 mL of a drug which has a strength of 25 mg/mL. How many mg will be administered?

Units of the answer	mg
Given	5 mL
Ratio(s) as stated	25 mg/mL
Ratios(s) as used	25 mg/mL

$$5 \text{ mL} \left(\frac{25 \text{ mg}}{\text{mL}}\right) = 125 \text{ mg}$$

10) A prescriber has ordered 375 mg of a drug which comes in a strength of 75 mg/mL. How many mL will be administered?

Units of the answer	mL
Given	375 mg
Ratio(s) as stated	75 mg/mL
Ratios(s) as used	1 mL/75 mg

$$375 \text{ mg} \left(\frac{1 \text{ mL}}{75 \text{ mg}}\right) = 5 \text{ mL}$$

Dosage Exercise Set 2 Answers

1) A patient is to receive 150 mg of a drug per day divided into 3 equal doses. The drug is available in 10 mL vials of 10 mg/mL. How many mL will be administered for each dose?

$$\left(\frac{150 \text{ mg}}{\text{day}}\right)\left(\frac{1 \text{ day}}{3 \text{ doses}}\right)\left(\frac{1 \text{ mL}}{10 \text{ mg}}\right) = \frac{5 \text{ mL}}{\text{dose}}$$

2) A patient who weighs 185 lb is to receive a dosage of 2 mg/kg/day for 4 days. The drug is available in 10 mL vials of 50 mg/mL. How many total mL will be administered over the 4 days.

$$185 \text{ lb} \left(\frac{1 \text{ kg}}{2.2 \text{ lb}}\right)\left(\frac{2 \text{ mg}}{\text{kg day}}\right)\left(\frac{4 \text{ days}}{1}\right)\left(\frac{1 \text{ mL}}{50 \text{ mg}}\right) = 13.5 \text{ mL}$$

3) A patient is ordered 600 mg/day in 4 equal doses. The drug is available in 10 mL vials of 50 mg/mL. How many mL will the patient receive in 1 dose?

$$\frac{600 \text{ mg}}{\text{day}}\left(\frac{1 \text{ day}}{4 \text{ doses}}\right)\left(\frac{1 \text{ mL}}{50 \text{ mg}}\right) = \frac{3 \text{ mL}}{\text{dose}}$$

4) A patient is prescribed 250 mg 3 times daily for 10 days. The drug is available in 125 mg capsules. How many capsules will be administered per dose?

Dosage Calculations for Nursing Students

$$\left(\frac{250 \text{ mg}}{\text{dose}}\right)\left(\frac{1 \text{ capsule}}{125 \text{ mg}}\right) = \frac{2 \text{ capsules}}{\text{dose}}$$

5) An 80 kg patient is prescribed 3 mg/kg/day for 7 days. The drug is available in 5 mL vials of 50 mg/mL. How many vials will be needed for the 7 days? Tip: Convert 3 mg/kg/day to 3 mg/(kg*day).

$$80 \text{ kg}\left(\frac{3 \text{ mg}}{\text{kg day}}\right)\left(\frac{1 \text{ mL}}{50 \text{ mg}}\right)\left(\frac{7 \text{ days}}{1}\right)\left(\frac{1 \text{ vial}}{5 \text{ mL}}\right) = 6.7 \text{ vials rounded up to 7 vials}$$

6) A patient is to receive 5 mL of a drug 3 times daily for 10 days. The drug is available in a strength of 25 mg/mL in a bottle of 240 mL. How many mg will the patient receive in each dose?

$$5 \text{ mL}\left(\frac{25 \text{ mg}}{\text{mL}}\right) = 125 \text{ mg}$$

7) A patient weighs 205 lbs and is prescribed a dosage of 600 mg IV given over 2 hours. The drug is available in 10 mL vials of 100 mg/ mL. How many mL will be administered?

$$600 \text{ mg}\left(\frac{1 \text{ mL}}{100 \text{ mg}}\right) = 6 \text{ mL}$$

8) A patient is to receive a dosage of 34 mg/kg/day each day for 60 days. The patient weighs 196 lb. The drug is available in 20 mL vials of 200 mg/mL. How many vials will be required for the 60 day course of therapy?

$$\frac{34 \text{ mg}}{\text{kg day}}\left(\frac{196 \text{ lb}}{1}\right)\left(\frac{1 \text{ kg}}{2.2 \text{ lb}}\right)\left(\frac{60 \text{ days}}{1}\right)\left(\frac{1 \text{ mL}}{200 \text{ mg}}\right)\left(\frac{1 \text{ vial}}{20 \text{ mL}}\right) = 45.4 \text{ vials rounded to 46 vials}$$

9) A patient is prescribed 250 mg 4 times daily. The drug is available in 125 mg capsules. How many capsules will be administered each day?

$$\left(\frac{250 \text{ mg}}{\text{dose}}\right)\left(\frac{4 \text{ doses}}{\text{day}}\right)\left(\frac{1 \text{ cap}}{125 \text{ mg}}\right) = \frac{8 \text{ caps}}{\text{day}}$$

10) Order: 25 mcg/kg/day divided into 4 equal doses. The patient's weight is 176 lb. The drug is available in 10 mL vials of 250 mcg/mL. How many mL will be administered for each dose?

$$\frac{25 \text{ mcg}}{\text{kg day}}\left(\frac{1 \text{ day}}{4 \text{ doses}}\right)\left(\frac{176 \text{ lb}}{1}\right)\left(\frac{1 \text{ kg}}{2.2 \text{ lb}}\right)\left(\frac{1 \text{ mL}}{250 \text{ mcg}}\right) = \frac{2 \text{ mL}}{\text{dose}}$$

IV Flow Rate Exercise Answers

Calculate the flow rate in mL/h.

1) 1000 mL infused over 5 h.

$$\frac{1000 \text{ mL}}{5 \text{ h}} = \frac{200 \text{ mL}}{\text{h}}$$

2) 250 mL infused over 2 h.

$$\frac{250 \text{ mL}}{2 \text{ h}} = \frac{125 \text{ mL}}{\text{h}}$$

Calculate the flow rate in gtts/min. Round to the nearest drop.

3) 1000 mL infused over 4 hours using an infusion set with a drop factor of 10 (10 gtts/mL).

$$\frac{1000 \text{ mL}}{4 \text{ h}} \left(\frac{10 \text{ gtts}}{\text{mL}}\right)\left(\frac{1 \text{ h}}{60 \text{ min}}\right) = \frac{42 \text{ gtts}}{\text{min}}$$

4) 250 mL infused over 2 hours using an infusion set with a drop factor of 15.

$$\frac{250 \text{ mL}}{2 \text{ h}} \left(\frac{15 \text{ gtts}}{\text{mL}}\right)\left(\frac{1 \text{ h}}{60 \text{ min}}\right) = \frac{31 \text{ gtts}}{\text{min}}$$

5) 2 L infused over 24 hours using an infusion set with a drop factor of 20.

$$\frac{2 \text{ L}}{24 \text{ h}}\left(\frac{1000 \text{ mL}}{\text{L}}\right)\left(\frac{20 \text{ gtts}}{\text{mL}}\right)\left(\frac{1 \text{ h}}{60 \text{ min}}\right) = \frac{28 \text{ gtts}}{\text{min}}$$

6) 100 mL infused over 1 hour using an infusion set with a drop factor of 10.

$$\frac{100 \text{ mL}}{1 \text{ h}}\left(\frac{10 \text{ gtts}}{\text{mL}}\right)\left(\frac{1 \text{ h}}{60 \text{ min}}\right) = \frac{17 \text{ gtts}}{\text{min}}$$

7) 1000 mL infused over 5 hours using an infusion set with a drop factor of 20.

$$\frac{1000 \text{ mL}}{5 \text{ h}}\left(\frac{20 \text{ gtts}}{\text{mL}}\right)\left(\frac{1 \text{ h}}{60 \text{ min}}\right) = \frac{67 \text{ gtts}}{\text{min}}$$

Calculate the length of time required to infuse the following volumes.

8) A 1000 mL bag infused at the rate of 45 mL/h.

$$1000 \text{ mL}\left(\frac{1 \text{ h}}{45 \text{ mL}}\right) = 22.2 \text{ h}$$

9) A 1000 mL bag infused at the rate of 45 mL/h using an infusion set with a drop factor of 20.

$$1000 \text{ mL}\left(\frac{1 \text{ h}}{45 \text{ mL}}\right) = 22.2 \text{ h}$$

10) A 1000 mL bag infused at the rate of 45 mL/h using an infusion set with a drop factor of 10.

$$1000 \text{ mL}\left(\frac{1 \text{ h}}{45 \text{ mL}}\right) = 22.2 \text{ h}$$

11) A 1 L bag infused at the rate of 50 gtts/min using an infusion set with a drop factor of 15.

$$1 \text{ L}\left(\frac{1000 \text{ mL}}{\text{L}}\right)\left(\frac{15 \text{ gtts}}{\text{mL}}\right)\left(\frac{1 \text{ min}}{50 \text{ gtts}}\right)\left(\frac{1 \text{ h}}{60 \text{ min}}\right) = 5 \text{ h}$$

Dosage Calculations for Nursing Students

12) A 500 mL bag infused at the rate of 25 gtts/min using an infusion set with a drop factor of 20.

$$500 \text{ mL} \left(\frac{20 \text{ gtts}}{\text{mL}}\right)\left(\frac{1 \text{ min}}{25 \text{ gtts}}\right)\left(\frac{1 \text{ h}}{60 \text{ min}}\right) = 6.7 \text{ h}$$

Answer the following. Round to the nearest drop or mL.

13) A patient has an order for regular insulin at the rate of 18 units/hour. The solution is 100 mL with 100 units of regular insulin. An infusion set with a drop factor of 20 is being used. What will be the flow rate in gtts/min? What is the flow rate in mL/h?

$$\frac{18 \text{ units}}{\text{h}}\left(\frac{100 \text{ mL}}{100 \text{ units}}\right)\left(\frac{20 \text{ gtts}}{\text{mL}}\right)\left(\frac{1 \text{ h}}{60 \text{ min}}\right) = \frac{6 \text{ gtts}}{\text{min}}$$

$$\frac{18 \text{ units}}{\text{h}}\left(\frac{100 \text{ mL}}{100 \text{ units}}\right) = \frac{18 \text{ mL}}{\text{h}}$$

14) A patient has an order for a drug to be infused at the rate of 5 mcg/kg/min. A 500 mL bag contains 250 mg of the drug and the patient weighs 185 pounds. An infusion set with a drop factor of 20 is being used. What is the flow rate in gtts/min? What is the flow rate in mL/h?

$$\frac{5 \text{ mcg}}{\text{kg min}}\left(\frac{185 \text{ lb}}{1}\right)\left(\frac{1 \text{ kg}}{2.2 \text{ lb}}\right)\left(\frac{500 \text{ mL}}{250 \text{ mg}}\right)\left(\frac{1 \text{ mg}}{1000 \text{ mcg}}\right)\left(\frac{20 \text{ gtts}}{\text{mL}}\right) = \frac{17 \text{ gtts}}{\text{min}}$$

$$\frac{5 \text{ mcg}}{\text{kg min}}\left(\frac{185 \text{ lb}}{1}\right)\left(\frac{1 \text{ kg}}{2.2 \text{ lb}}\right)\left(\frac{500 \text{ mL}}{250 \text{ mg}}\right)\left(\frac{1 \text{ mg}}{1000 \text{ mcg}}\right)\left(\frac{60 \text{ min}}{\text{h}}\right) = \frac{50 \text{ mL}}{\text{h}}$$

15) A patient has an order for a drug to be infused at the rate of 25 mg/kg/h. A 1 L bag contains 10 g of the drug and the patient weighs 80 kg. An infusion set with a drop factor of 15 is being used. What is the flow rate in gtts/min? What is the flow rate in mL/h?

$$\left(\frac{25 \text{ mg}}{\text{kg h}}\right)\left(\frac{80 \text{ kg}}{1}\right)\left(\frac{1 \text{ h}}{60 \text{ min}}\right)\left(\frac{1 \text{ L}}{10 \text{ g}}\right)\left(\frac{1000 \text{ mL}}{\text{L}}\right)\left(\frac{1 \text{ g}}{1000 \text{ mg}}\right)\left(\frac{15 \text{ gtts}}{\text{mL}}\right) = \frac{50 \text{ gtts}}{\text{min}}$$

$$\left(\frac{25 \text{ mg}}{\text{kg h}}\right)\left(\frac{80 \text{ kg}}{1}\right)\left(\frac{1 \text{ L}}{10 \text{ g}}\right)\left(\frac{1000 \text{ mL}}{\text{L}}\right)\left(\frac{1 \text{ g}}{1000 \text{ mg}}\right) = \frac{200 \text{ mL}}{\text{h}}$$

In practice, you would probably change the 1 L bag to 1000 mL and the 10 g to 10,000 mg before you started the problem. This would simplify things a bit and result with the following calculations.

$$\left(\frac{25 \text{ mg}}{\text{kg h}}\right)\left(\frac{80 \text{ kg}}{1}\right)\left(\frac{1 \text{ h}}{60 \text{ min}}\right)\left(\frac{1000 \text{ mL}}{10,000 \text{ mg}}\right)\left(\frac{15 \text{ gtts}}{\text{mL}}\right) = \frac{50 \text{ gtts}}{\text{min}}$$

$$\left(\frac{25 \text{ mg}}{\text{kg h}}\right)\left(\frac{80 \text{ kg}}{1}\right)\left(\frac{1000 \text{ mL}}{10,000 \text{ mg}}\right) = \frac{200 \text{ mL}}{\text{h}}$$

Percent Exercise Answers

1) Convert the following numbers to percents using the format in the examples below.

0.35	(0.35)(100%)=35%
15/17	(15/17)(100%)=88.24%
0.98	(0.98)(100%)=98%
1.78	(1.78)(100%)=178%
3.99	(3.99)(100%) = 399%
0.05	(0.05)(100%)=5%
0.003	(0.003)(100%)=0.3%
1.25	(1.25)(100%)=125%
6/9	(6/9)(100%)=66.7%
5.45	(5.45)(100%)=545%
9.95	(9.95)(100%)=995%
0.005	(0.005)(100%)=0.5%

2) Convert the following percents to numbers using the format in the example below.

56%	$\frac{56\%}{100\%} = 0.56$
3.5%	$\frac{3.5\%}{100\%} = 0.035$
99%	$\frac{99\%}{100\%} = 0.99$
101%	$\frac{101\%}{100\%} = 1.01$
34.5%	$\frac{34.5\%}{100\%} = 0.345$
85.67%	$\frac{85.67\%}{100\%} = 0.8567$
3.35%	$\frac{3.35\%}{100\%} = 0.0335$
3%	$\frac{3\%}{100\%} = 0.03$

Dosage Calculations for Nursing Students

Percent Change Exercise Answers

For the following calculate the percent change and indicate if it is an increase or decrease.

1) A patient's weight is 171 lb. on Monday and 173 lb. on Thursday.

$$\frac{173 \text{ lb} - 171 \text{ lb}}{171 \text{ lb}}(100\%) = \frac{2 \text{ lb}}{171 \text{ lb}}(100\%) = 1.2\% \text{ (increase)}$$

2) A patient weighs 192 lb. on Wednesday and one week later weighs 85 kg.

$$\frac{85 \text{ kg} - 87.3 \text{ kg}}{87.3 \text{ kg}}(100\%) = \frac{-2.3 \text{ kg}}{87.3 \text{ kg}}(100\%) = -2.6\% \text{ (decrease)}$$

3) A drug is dosed at 5 mcg/kg/min then increased to 6.2 mcg/kg/min.

$$\frac{6.2 \text{ mcg} - 5 \text{ mcg}}{5 \text{ mcg}}(100\%) = \frac{1.2 \text{ mcg}}{5 \text{ mcg}}(100\%) = 24\% \text{ (increase}$$

4) You got a merit raise in pay from $48.75 per hour to $50.00 per hour.

$$\frac{\$50.00 - \$48.75}{\$48.75}(100\%) = \frac{\$1.25}{\$48.75}(100\%) = 2.6\% \text{ (increase)}$$

Percent Strength Exercise Answers

Express the following as percent strength solution, and include the type of solution (w/w, w/v, v/v).

1) 7 g KCl in 200 mL

$$\frac{7 \text{ g}}{200 \text{ mL}}(100\%) = 3.5\% \frac{\text{g}}{\text{mL}} = 3.5\% \frac{\text{w}}{\text{v}}$$

2) 3.5 g NaCl in 1000 mL

$$\frac{3.5 \text{ g}}{1000 \text{ mL}}(100\%) = 0.35\% \frac{\text{g}}{\text{mL}} = 0.35\% \frac{\text{w}}{\text{v}}$$

3) 7.9 mg NaHCO$_3$ in 100 mL

$$\frac{7.9 \text{ mg}}{100 \text{ mL}}\left(\frac{1 \text{ g}}{1000 \text{ mg}}\right)(100\%) = 0.0079\% \frac{\text{g}}{\text{mL}} = 0.0079\% \frac{\text{w}}{\text{v}}$$

4) 5 mcg NaCl in 0.25 mL

$$\frac{5 \text{ mcg}}{0.25 \text{ mL}}\left(\frac{1 \text{ mg}}{1000 \text{ mcg}}\right)\left(\frac{1 \text{ g}}{1000 \text{ mg}}\right)(100\%) = 0.002\% \frac{\text{g}}{\text{mL}} = 0.002\% \frac{\text{w}}{\text{v}}$$

5) 45 g NaCl in 3 L

$$\frac{45 \text{ g}}{3 \text{ L}}\left(\frac{1 \text{ L}}{1000 \text{ mL}}\right)(100\%) = 1.5\% \frac{\text{g}}{\text{mL}} = 1.5\% \frac{\text{w}}{\text{v}}$$

6) 3 g HC in 200 g HC ointment

$$\frac{3 \text{ g}}{200 \text{ g}}(100\%) = 1.5\% \frac{\text{g}}{\text{g}} = 1.5\% \frac{\text{w}}{\text{w}}$$

7) 5 g coal tar in 300 g coal tar ointment

Dosage Calculations for Nursing Students

$$\frac{5\text{ g}}{300\text{ g}}(100\%) = 1.7\% \frac{g}{g} = 1.7\% \frac{w}{w}$$

8) 5 mg betamethasone in 10 g betamethasone ointment

$$\frac{5\text{ mg}}{10\text{ g}}\left(\frac{1\text{ g}}{1000\text{ mg}}\right)(100\%) = 0.05\% \frac{g}{g} = 0.05\% \frac{w}{w}$$

9) 20 g urea in 40 g urea ointment

$$\frac{20\text{ g}}{40\text{ g}}(100\%) = 50\% \frac{g}{g} = 50\% \frac{w}{w}$$

10) 18 g salicylic acid in 300 g salicylic acid cream

$$\frac{18\text{ g}}{300\text{ g}}(100\%) = 6\% \frac{g}{g} = 6\% \frac{w}{w}$$

11) 900 mL IPA in 1000 mL IPA solution

$$\frac{900\text{ mL}}{1000\text{ mL}}(100\%) = 90\% \frac{mL}{mL} = 90\% \frac{v}{v}$$

12) 40 mL ETOH in 100 mL ETOH solution

$$\frac{40\text{ mL}}{100\text{ mL}}(100\%) = 40\% \frac{mL}{mL} = 40\% \frac{v}{v}$$

Answer the following:

13) How many mg of NaCl are in 10 mL of 0.9% NaCl (normal saline).

$$10\text{ mL}\left(\frac{0.9\%\text{ g}}{mL}\right)\left(\frac{1}{100\%}\right)\left(\frac{1000\text{ mg}}{g}\right) = 90\text{ mg}$$

Note: It is easier to just write 100% under the 0.9% g rather than multiply by $\left(\frac{1}{100\%}\right)$, so the following problems will be in that format.

14) How many g of NaCl are in 2 L of NS (Normal Saline)

$$2\text{ L}\left(\frac{0.9\%\text{ g}}{100\%\text{ mL}}\right)\left(\frac{1000\text{ mL}}{L}\right) = 18\text{ g}$$

15) How many g of KCl are in 473 mL of 20% KCl?

$$473\text{ mL}\left(\frac{20\%\text{ g}}{100\%\text{ mL}}\right) = 94.6\text{ g}$$

16) How many mg of bupivacaine are in 30 mL of 0.5% bupivacaine solution?

$$30\text{ mL}\left(\frac{0.5\%\text{ g}}{100\%\text{ mL}}\right)\left(\frac{1000\text{ mg}}{g}\right) = 150\text{ mg}$$

17) How many mg of lidocaine are in 100 mL of 1% lidocaine?

$$100\text{ mL}\left(\frac{1\%\text{ g}}{100\%\text{ mL}}\right)\left(\frac{1000\text{ mg}}{g}\right) = 1000\text{ mg}$$

18) How many mcg of NaCl are in 1 drop of 0.9% NaCl if there are 20 drops/mL?

$$1\text{ drop}\left(\frac{1\text{ mL}}{20\text{ drops}}\right)\left(\frac{0.9\%\text{ g}}{100\%\text{ mL}}\right)\left(\frac{1000\text{ mg}}{g}\right)\left(\frac{1000\text{ mcg}}{mg}\right) = 450\text{ mcg}$$

Dosage Calculations for Nursing Students

19) How many mL of ETOH are in 60 mL of 80 proof (40% ETOH) tequila?

$$60 \text{ mL} \left(\frac{40\% \text{ mL}}{100\% \text{ mL}}\right) = 24 \text{ mL}$$

20) How many g of HC are in 500 g of 2.5% HC ointment?

$$500 \text{ g} \left(\frac{2.5\% \text{ g}}{100\% \text{ g}}\right) = 12.5 \text{ g}$$

Ratio Strength Exercise Answers

1) How many grams of active ingredient are in 500 mL of a 1:10,000 solution?

$$500 \text{ mL} \left(\frac{1 \text{ g}}{10,000 \text{ mL}}\right) = 0.05 \text{ g}$$

2) How many grams of active ingredient are in 40 mL of a 1:200 solution?

$$40 \text{ mL} \left(\frac{1 \text{ g}}{200 \text{ mL}}\right) = 0.2 \text{ g}$$

3) How many grams of active ingredient are in 600 g of a 1:25 w/w preparation?

$$600 \text{ g prep} \left(\frac{1 \text{ g AI}}{25 \text{ g prep}}\right) = 24 \text{ g AI}$$

4) How many mg of active ingredient are in 800 mL of a 1:10,000 solution?

$$800 \text{ mL} \left(\frac{1 \text{ g}}{10,000 \text{ mL}}\right)\left(\frac{1000 \text{ mg}}{\text{g}}\right) = 80 \text{ mg}$$

5) How many mcg are in 10 mL of a 1:100,000 solution?

$$10 \text{ mL} \left(\frac{1 \text{ g}}{100,000 \text{ mL}}\right)\left(\frac{1000 \text{ mg}}{\text{g}}\right)\left(\frac{1000 \text{ mcg}}{\text{mg}}\right) = 100 \text{ mcg}$$

6) You have a 10 mL vial which is labeled 1:10,000 and you are asked to draw up 0.4 mg of drug. How many mL would you draw?

$$0.4 \text{ mg} \left(\frac{10,000 \text{ mL}}{1 \text{ g}}\right)\left(\frac{1 \text{ g}}{1000 \text{ mg}}\right) = 4 \text{ mL}$$

7) You have a 50 mL vial which is labeled 1:1000 and are asked to draw up 1 mg. How many mL would you draw?

$$1 \text{ mg} \left(\frac{1000 \text{ mL}}{1 \text{ g}}\right)\left(\frac{1 \text{ g}}{1000 \text{ mg}}\right) = 1 \text{ mL}$$

8) You have a solution which is 1:10,000 w/v. What is the percentage strength?

$$\left(\frac{1 \text{ g}}{10,000 \text{ mL}}\right) 100\% = 0.01\% \frac{\text{g}}{\text{mL}} = 0.01\% \frac{\text{w}}{\text{v}}$$

9) What is the percentage strength of a 1:100 w/v solution?

$$\left(\frac{1 \text{ g}}{100 \text{ mL}}\right) 100\% = 1\% \frac{\text{g}}{\text{mL}} = 1\% \frac{\text{w}}{\text{v}}$$

10) You have a 100 mL vial which is labeled 1:1000. How many mg are in 25 mL of the solution?

$$25 \text{ mL} \left(\frac{1 \text{ g}}{1000 \text{ mL}}\right)\left(\frac{1000 \text{ mg}}{\text{g}}\right) = 25 \text{ mg}$$

Dosage Calculations for Nursing Students

Milliequivalent Exercise Answers

1) Look up the atomic masses (atomic weights) of the following elements.

Name	Atomic Symbol	Atomic Mass (rounded to nearest tenth)	Ionic Form
Hydrogen	H	1.0	H^+ (Hydrogen Ion)
Carbon	C	12.0	
Oxygen	O	16.0	
Sodium	Na	23.0	Na^+ (Sodium Ion)
Magnesium	Mg	24.3	Mg^{++} (Magnesium Ion)
Chlorine	Cl	35.5	Cl^- (Chloride Ion)
Potassium	K	39.1	K^+ (Potassium Ion)
Calcium	Ca	40.1	Ca^{++} (Calcium Ion)
Sulfur	S	32.1	

2) Now that you know the atomic masses of each of the elements, fill in the formula masses of the listed polyatomic ions (ions with more than one atom). Add up all the individual masses. CH_3COO^- has two carbons atoms, three hydrogen atoms, and two oxygen atoms.

Name	Chemical Formula	Formula Mass	Ionic Form
Acetate	CH_3COO^-	59.0	CH_3COO^-
Bicarbonate	HCO_3^-	61.0	HCO_3^-
Sulfate	SO_4^{-2}	96.1	SO_4^{2-}

3) List the formula masses of the following ionic compounds.

Name	Chemical Formula	Formula Mass	Ionic Form
Sodium Chloride	NaCl	58.5	$Na^+ Cl^-$
Potassium Chloride	KCl	74.6	$K^+ Cl^-$
Calcium Chloride	$CaCl_2$	111.1	$Ca^{++} 2Cl^-$
Magnesium Chloride	$MgCl_2$	95.3	$Mg^{++} 2Cl^-$
Sodium Acetate	CH_3COONa	82.0	$Na^+ CH_3COO^-$
Potassium Acetate	CH_3COOK	98.1	$K^+ CH_3COO^-$
Magnesium Sulfate	$MgSO_4$	120.4	$Mg^{++} SO_4^{2-}$
Sodium Bicarbonate	$NaHCO_3$	84.0	$Na^+ HCO_3^-$

4) Fill in the table with the ratios of mg/mmol and mEq/mmol for each compound.

Name	Chemical Formula	mg/mmol (ratio)	mEq/mmol (ratio)
Sodium Chloride	NaCl	58.5 mg/mmol	1 mEq/mmol
Potassium Chloride	KCl	74.6 mg/mmol	1 mEq/mmol
Calcium Chloride	$CaCl_2$	111.1 mg/mmol	2 mEq/mmol
Magnesium Chloride	$MgCl_2$	95.3 mg/mmol	2 mEq/mmol
Sodium Acetate	CH_3COONa	82.0 mg/mmol	1 mEq/mmol
Potassium Acetate	CH_3COOK	98.1 mg/mmol	1 mEq/mmol
Magnesium Sulfate	$MgSO_4$	120.4 mg/mmol	2 mEq/mmol
Sodium Bicarbonate	$NaHCO_3$	84.0 mg/mmol	1 mEq/mmol

Dosage Calculations for Nursing Students

5) How many mEq are contained in 746 mg of KCl?

$$746 \text{ mg} \left(\frac{1 \text{ mmol}}{74.6 \text{ mg}}\right)\left(\frac{1 \text{ mEq}}{\text{mmol}}\right) = 10 \text{ mEq}$$

Note: In this case where there is 1 mEq per mmol, you can skip the extra step of including the $\left(\frac{1 \text{ mEq}}{\text{mmol}}\right)$ conversion factor and just use $\left(\frac{1 \text{ mEq}}{74.6 \text{ mg}}\right)$.

6) How many mEq of calcium chloride are contained in 2 g of calcium chloride?

$$2 \text{ g}\left(\frac{1 \text{ mmol}}{111.1 \text{ mg}}\right)\left(\frac{2 \text{ mEq}}{\text{mmol}}\right)\left(\frac{1000 \text{ mg}}{\text{g}}\right) = 36 \text{ mEq}$$

7) How many mEq of Ca^{++} are in 2 g of calcium chloride?

This is the same as problem #6. If there are 36 mEq of $CaCl_2$, there are 36 mEq of Ca^{++} and 36 mEq of Cl^-.

8) How many mg of magnesium sulfate are in 10 mEq of magnesium sulfate?

$$10 \text{ mEq}\left(\frac{120.4 \text{ mg}}{\text{mmol}}\right)\left(\frac{1 \text{ mmol}}{2 \text{ mEq}}\right) = 602 \text{ mg}$$

9) How many g of sodium acetate are in 12 mEq of sodium acetate?

$$12 \text{ mEq}\left(\frac{82.0 \text{ mg}}{\text{mEq}}\right)\left(\frac{1 \text{ g}}{1000 \text{ mg}}\right) = 0.984 \text{ g}$$

10) How many mEq of NaCl are in 2 L of 0.9% NaCl?

$$2 \text{ L}\left(\frac{0.9\% \text{ g}}{\text{ml}}\right)\left(\frac{1}{100\%}\right)\left(\frac{1000 \text{ mg}}{\text{g}}\right)\left(\frac{1000 \text{ ml}}{\text{L}}\right)\left(\frac{1 \text{ mEq}}{58.5 \text{ mg}}\right) = 307.7 \text{ mEq}$$

11) How many mEq of KCl are in 30 mL of 10% KCl solution?

$$30 \text{ mL}\left(\frac{10\% \text{ g}}{\text{mL}}\right)\left(\frac{1}{100\%}\right)\left(\frac{1000 \text{ mg}}{\text{g}}\right)\left(\frac{1 \text{ mEq}}{74.6 \text{ mg}}\right) = 40.2 \text{ mEq}$$

12) How many mEq of $MgSO_4$ are contained in 10 g of $MgSO_4$?

$$10 \text{ g}\left(\frac{1 \text{ mmol}}{120.4 \text{ mg}}\right)\left(\frac{2 \text{ mEq}}{\text{mmol}}\right)\left(\frac{1000 \text{ mg}}{\text{g}}\right) = 166.1 \text{ mEq}$$

13) How many mg of Na^+ (just the sodium) are contained in 1.5 L of 10% NaCl?

$$1.5 \text{ L}\left(\frac{10\% \text{ g}}{\text{ml}}\right)\left(\frac{1}{100\%}\right)\left(\frac{1000 \text{ mg}}{\text{g}}\right)\left(\frac{1000 \text{ ml}}{\text{L}}\right) = 150,000 \text{ mg NaCl}$$

Since the ratio of the weight of sodium (Na^+) to the weight of sodium chloride (NaCl) is $\frac{23.0 \text{ mg Na+}}{58.5 \text{ mg NaCl}}$ (from the atomic masses):

$$150,000 \text{ mg NaCl}\left(\frac{23.0 \text{ mg Na}^+}{58.5 \text{ mg NaCl}}\right) = 58,974 \text{ mg Na}^+$$

14) Try this one if you wish. You have 2.5 L of 10% NaCl solution and your friend has 1.5 L of $MgSO_4$ solution. You have twice as many mEq of NaCl as your friend has of mEq of $MgSO_4$. What is the percentage strength of your friend's $MgSO_4$?

Step 1) Figure out how many mEq of NaCl you have.

$$2.5 \text{ L} \left(\frac{10\% \text{ g}}{\text{ml}}\right)\left(\frac{1}{100\%}\right)\left(\frac{1000 \text{ mg}}{\text{g}}\right)\left(\frac{1000 \text{ ml}}{\text{L}}\right)\left(\frac{1 \text{ mEq}}{58.5 \text{ mg}}\right) = 4{,}273.5 \text{ mEq NaCl}$$

Step 2) You know that you have twice as many mEq of NaCl as your friend has mEq of MgSO$_4$, so your friend would have 2,136.8 mEq of MgSO$_4$. Now change the 2,136.8 mEq into g.

$$2{,}136.8 \text{ mEq} \left(\frac{1 \text{ mmol}}{2 \text{ mEq}}\right)\left(\frac{120.4 \text{ mg}}{\text{mmol}}\right)\left(\frac{1 \text{ g}}{1000 \text{ mg}}\right) = 128.6 \text{ g MgSO}_4$$

Step 3) Now you know how many g of MgSO$_4$ and how many mL of solution your friend has, so you just have to convert that into a percent strength.

$$\frac{128.6 \text{ g}}{1.5 \text{ L}}(100\%)\left(\frac{1 \text{ L}}{1000 \text{ mL}}\right) = 8.57\% \frac{\text{g}}{\text{mL}} = 8.57\% \frac{\text{w}}{\text{v}}$$

Dosage Calculations for Nursing Students

Self-Assessment Exercise Answers

Part 1:

Convert the following (1 point each):

1) 1.1 L to mL **1100 mL**

2) 3.2 cm to mm **32 mm**

3) 60 mcg to mg **0.06 mg**

4) 200 mcg to mg **0.2 mg**

5) 2.2 kg to lb **4.8 lb**

6) 145 lb to kg **65.9 kg**

7) 30 mL to tsp **6 tsp**

8) 130 mg to gr **2 gr**

9) 1 fl oz to tbs **2 tbs**

10) 160 lb to kg **72.7 kg**

Round the following to the nearest tenth (1 point each):

11) 16.59 mg **16.6 mg**

12) 20.179 mg **20.2 mg**

13) 1.43 L **1.4 L**

14) What is the Roman numeral for 5? (1 point) **V**

15) What is the Roman numeral for 4? (1 point) **IV**

Convert the following times (1 point each):

16) 1:05 PM to military time. **1305**

17) 12:07 AM to military time. **0007**

18) 1430 to civilian time. **2:30 PM**

19-30: Calculate the amount to administer and round to the nearest tenth. 2 points each.

19)

Order	150 mg IM
Available	300 mg/mL
Administer	**0.5 mL**

20)

Order	600 mg IV
Available	1 g/10 mL
Administer	**0.6 mL**

21)

Order	500 mg PO
Available	250 mg tab
Administer	**2 tabs**

22)

Order	10 mg IV
Available	5 mg/mL
Administer	**2 mL**

23)

Order	2 mg/kg
Available	40 mg/mL
Pt Weight	62 kg
Administer	**3.1 mL**

24)

Order	5 mg/kg
Available	80 mg/mL
Pt Weight	190 lb
Administer	**5.4 mL**

25)

Order	1 mg/kg
Available	40 mg/mL
Pt Weight	176 lb
Administer	**2 mL**

26)

Order	5 mcg/kg
Available	30 mcg/mL
Pt Weight	12 kg
Administer	**2 mL**

27)

Order	8 mcg/kg
Available	100 mcg/mL
Pt Weight	126 lb
Administer	**4.6 mL**

28)

Order	6 mcg/kg/day divided into 4 equal doses.
Available	100 mcg/mL
Pt Weight	175 lb
Administer/dose	**1.2 mL**

29)

Order	2 mg/kg/day divided into 2 equal doses
Available	25 mg/mL
Pt Weight	120 lb
Administer/dose	**2.2 mL**

30)

Order	10 mg/kg/day divided into 3 equal doses
Available	20 mg/mL
Pt Weight	14 kg
Administer	**2.3 mL**

Dosage Calculations for Nursing Students

31-36: Calculate the following flow rates in mL/h. Round to the nearest mL. (2 points each)

31) Infuse 1500 mL over 6 hours. **250 mL/h**

32) Infuse 1000 mL over 4 hours 30 min. **222 mL/h**

33) Infuse 250 mL over 5 hours. **50 mL/h**

34-36: Calculate the following flow rates in gtts/min. (2 points each)

34) Infuse 500 mL over 6 hours with a drop factor of 20 (20 gtts/mL). **28 gtts/min**

35) Infuse 1000 mL over 3 hours 15 min with a drop factor of 10. **51 gtts/min**

36) Infuse 500 mL over 7 hours with a drop factor of 15. **18 gtts/min**

37) You have an order to start a Pitocin infusion at 5 mUnits/min. You have on hand a 100 mL bag containing 10 Units of Pitocin. At what rate will you set the IV pump in mL/h? Round to the nearest mL/h. (3 points) **3 mL/h**

38) You have an order to start a DOPamine infusion at the rate of 4 mcg/kg/min on a 185 lb patient. You have a DOPamine 800 mg in 500 mL D5W. At what rate will you set the IV pump in mL/h? Round to the nearest tenth mL/h. (3 points) **12.6 mL/h**

39) You have an order to start a DOBUTtamine infusion at the rate of 2 mcg/kg/min on a 160 lb patient. You have on hand 500 mg DOBUTamine in 250 mL D5W. At what rate will you set the IV pump in mL/h? Round to the nearest tenth mL/h. (3 points) **4.4 mL/h**

40-42: Convert each of the following decimal numbers into a percent. (1 point each)

40) 0.45 **45%**

41) 0.02 **2%**

42) 1.3 **130%**

43-45: Convert the following percents into decimal numbers. (1 point each)

43) 67% **0.67**

44) 32.1% **0.321**

45) 101% **1.01**

46) Your patient weighed 84 kg when admitted and now weighs 81 kg. What is the percent change to the nearest tenth of a percent? (2 points) **3.6%**

47) A patient's medication dosage went from 400 mg/day to 600 mg/day. What is the percent change to the nearest tenth of a percent? (2 points) **50%**

48) How many mcg of a drug are contained in 1 mL of a 1:10,000 solution? (2 points) **0.1 mg**

49) How many mg of NaCl are contained in 100 mL of 0.9% NaCl? (2 points) **900 mg**

50) A student is celebrating after finishing the dosage calculation class by drinking a margarita with 2 fl oz of 80 proof tequila in it. Proof is twice the percent v/v ethanol. How many mL of ethanol did she consume? (2 points) **24 mL**

End of Part 1. 79 total points possible. Calculate your percent score by dividing your total points by 79 then multiplying by 100%.

Dosage Calculations for Nursing Students

Part 2:

1-3: Convert the following (1 point each):

1) 302 ng to mg. **0.000302 mg**

2) 2.5 dL to mL **250 mL**

3) 2.4 ML to L. (Note: ML is NOT the same as mL). **2,400,000 L**

4-6: Write the following numbers in scientific notation (1 point each):

4) 0.000000682 **6.82 X 10^{-7}**

5) 0.0000000002955 **2.955 X 10^{-10}**

6) 1,590,000,000,000,000 **1.59 X 10^{15}**

7) T or F: A mEq of Na^+ weighs the same as a mEq of K^+. (1 point) **F**

8) How many mEq of calcium chloride are contained in 1.6 g of calcium chloride? (3 points) **28.8 mEq**

9) How many mEq of KCl are in 45 mL of 20% KCl solution? (3 points) **120.6 mEq**

10) How many mg of sodium acetate are in 10 mEq of sodium acetate? (3 points) **820 mg**

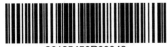

Made in the USA
San Bernardino, CA
16 February 2019